# GIFTED CHILDREN

for Hugh

# Gifted Children

Their Identification and Development
in a Social Context

by

JOAN FREEMAN

Director
The Gulbenkian Research Project on Gifted Children

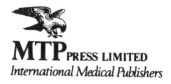
**MTP** PRESS LIMITED
*International Medical Publishers*

Published by
MTP Press Limited
Falcon House
Lancaster, England

Copyright © 1979   Joan Freeman
Paperback edition first published 1980

British Library Cataloguing in Publication Data

Freeman, Joan
   Gifted children.
   1.  Children – England
   2.  Gifted children
   I.  Title  II. Gulbenkian Research Project
   on Gifted Children
   301.43′14        HQ792.G7

   ISBN  0–85200–250–5 (hardback)
   ISBN  0–85200–375–7 (paperback)

Phototypesetting by Rainbow Graphics, Liverpool
Printed and bound in Great Britain by
Redwood Burn Limited
Trowbridge & Esher

# Contents

FOREWORD *by Sir Desmond Lee*     vii

ACKNOWLEDGEMENTS     ix

INTRODUCTION     xi

Chapter 1    MEANINGS OF GIFTEDNESS     1

*Giftedness is described in its social context. It is reviewed through history to the present day in these terms. The traditional mythic view of gifted children and their behaviour is examined. Scientific evidence is little, but even so it is often ignored. The effect of mythic thinking is considered in the identification of gifted children and the present interest in gifted children is examined.*

Chapter 2    LEARNING TO BE GIFTED     21

*Growing up in society; how a gifted child learns the social mores of the society in which it is born. Family influences are described and their resulting effects on the gifted child.*

Chapter 3    JUDGING GIFTEDNESS     71

*Physical and mental development of gifted children is discussed. Reference is made to early stimulation, nourishment, etc. A discussion is offered of what intelligence might be, and the controversy over its measurement. Research method and its problems are described.*

*v*

Chapter 4   THE GULBENKIAN PROJECT ON
            GIFTED CHILDREN                                        131

*A description of the 'Gulbenkian Project' is presented. This research
compared children who were labelled gifted with those who were not so
labelled but of equal ability, and a group of normal children. The research
was designed to find the behaviour and attitudes of the children, families
and schools. The perhaps controversial results are presented clearly and
briefly.*

Chapter 5   GIFTED CHILDREN IN PERSPECTIVE                        215

*The research is reviewed; conclusions are offered as to who are gifted
children and what brings them to notice. The problems of 'normal' gifted
children are described and how they may be coped with. Indications from
the research are presented as to how to educate gifted children. An outline is
given of types of special education which can be offered to them.*

            BIBLIOGRAPHY                                          281

            INDEX                                                 289

# Foreword

The concept of giftedness (unhappily perhaps so named) is a comparative newcomer to the educational scene. The work of Terman was of course known; IQ tests stalked the classroom and the slow and handicapped learner's problems were recognized. But it is only comparatively recently that the fast learner and the very clever have been recognized as having their problems too. That recognition has been not a little due to the work of the NAGC, to which all credit should be given for pressing for it when it was needed. We have therefore had in recent years many descriptions of the gifted child and his or her characteristics; but we are still rather short - and this is one of Joan Freeman's complaints - of rigorously conducted research. This project of hers has been carried out under the most rigorous requirements governing research of this kind, and though no project can answer all questions hers does make an important contribution to the subject. It has the further merit, in my opinion, that its conclusions confirm what the intelligent observer would expect. The target group of NAGC children *are* highly intelligent; the parents know their children. On the other hand a rather higher proportion of them have problems than those in the control group, which amounts to saying that parents consult NAGC if they have problems and not that gifted children are always problem children. Indeed, when gifted children do have problems these are due not to their being gifted but to causes which operate equally with all children. Of course, there are some problems and frustrations which particularly affect the gifted, but it is the business of schools to be aware of and deal with them; some schools no doubt do this better than others, but if the problems are recognized there is no call for separate and special schools. There may be some exceptions (e.g. music, with which Joan Freeman is not directly concerned) and some call for special treatment, but being gifted is not a disability. The gifted child is generally healthy and happy, and (as I well know) enormous fun to teach. He or she has, Joan Freeman finds, only one persistent fault – bad handwriting. Perhaps the mind moves too fast for the hand. We should be grateful to the NAGC and the Gulbenkian Foundation for enabling her to make this valuable contribution to the subject.

*Cambridge, 1979*                                    SIR DESMOND LEE

# Acknowledgements

I am indebted to many people for their kindness during the research and production of this book. It was Margaret Branch, a founder of the National Association for Gifted Children, who involved me in this research project and Henry Collis the present Director of the association who with encouragement and diplomacy enabled the work to proceed. Gillian Parker's sensitive research contribution was invaluable. Sir Desmond Lee's advice and support were more than welcome, as was Lady Lee's friendship. To the children, parents and teachers who gave so freely of their time and energy, I can only offer a sincere thankyou. My own children, Stephen, Justin, Felix and Rachel, were brave and uncomplaining throughout. David Bloomer, Managing Director of MTP, gave me the kind of support that other authors can only hope for. The exciting cover photograph by Harold Riley is greatly appreciated. But it is to Hugh, my husband, that I owe my deep gratitude for his steady, loving and very real help.

The research project and this book have been funded by The Calouste Gulbenkian Foundation. Peter Brinson, Director of the United Kingdom and Commonwealth Branch, and Millicent Bowerman, Literary Editor, have given me generous encouragement over the years.

JOAN FREEMAN

# Introduction

The identification of children who come to be termed gifted is a complex process. There is considerable difficulty in distinguishing the gifted child from those who are culturally fortunate. but of normal ability, and those who have all the 'symptoms' of giftedness, but achieve poorly.

There has recently been a rapidly growing interest in gifted children and a proliferation of groups for their benefit. This has been partly out of concern for the full growth of the potential of the individual child and partly with a view to the ability-power which would be available if such children were educated in a  suitable' way.

This book is a presentation of significant research into the problems of identifying gifted children within their social contexts. It begins with an explanation of gifted children in the context of social learning, that is how they and other children learn to live with other people. It goes on to consider the social contexts of psychological testing, what it is for and who it is for. Psychological testing is also considered from the point of view of its value as a measurement of present abilities, and as a predictive guide for gifted children.

The final part of the book is devoted to the author's research and to the conclusions reached on the basis of that evidence. Many of the results of the research are given throughout the text where they seem to be appropriate, but the work is described in full in Chapter 4. These findings are put into the perspective of other research findings on gifted children and of consideration for their education.

The book describes the first investigation of the gifted child in his or her own environment. It is not a comprehensive textbook of social psychology, but an outline of those aspects of the subject which are particularly relevant to the gifted child. Children are referred to as of either sex in the text, both to avoid the clumsy he/she, his/hers vocabulary and to extend the image of the psychological subject as being female, as well as the usual male. Although statistical evidence is offered in presenting the results of the research, the children are never regarded merely as sets of figures, but always as individual people.

CHAPTER 1

# Meanings of Giftedness

---

Because of the considerable confusion which surrounds the idea of giftedness, this chapter is concerned with the problems that arise in attempting to understand it – a theme which continues throughout the book. Different theories which might act as an aid towards placing giftedness in its cultural context are discussed here, though the influence of social factors in the development of gifted children is little understood as yet. There is a long way to go before these exceptional children can be universally recognized and catered for in an appropriate way.

Descriptions of giftedness are always based on the social values of the time and culture in which they are given. Throughout history, the meaning of giftedness has shifted according to the interests and preconceptions of people using the term and, like beauty, giftedness is often in the eye of the beholder. For example, at the height of the Roman Empire, a truly gifted man would be expected to conquer other nations, whereas a contemporary Roman might aim for the Nobel Peace Prize. Some Eastern countries consider the ability to go into a trance as a great gift, but in the West it is not generally valued in that way.

Although they are often used as if synonymous, it is necessary at the outset to differentiate between giftedness and achievement. To be gifted implies potential; achievement is the realization of potential. We cannot measure potential as such, but only measure achievement and judge potential from that. The current use of the term 'gifted child' is not based on any absolute criteria, but that is not to say that the definition is thereby spurious. It is important to realize, though, that there are motives, which are not always conscious or given recognition, underlying the choice of such a description. Motives come from a variety of sources, and these may appear to others as honourable, selfish or mistaken, according to their points of view.

Today, the term 'gifted' is used both to describe an all-round high level of ability in children, and specific abilities; it is therefore a relative concept. Even in the same field of activity, children are called gifted at different levels of achievement. In some schools, it is used to describe a child's high performance in relation to that of the rest of the children in that particular school, which may be poor. In the same way, some children in highly selective schools who are regarded as unintelligent in relation to their schoolmates would be considered gifted in another school. In some American states, children of ethnic or deprived minorities are not now measured on the same tests as culturally more fortunate children, since their performance on these, for whatever reasons, have not always been as good (Jensen, 1973a). But using different tests, a child who would have scored badly on a conventional intelligence test can now be considered gifted on a specially designed one. Thus the value of the term gifted can only be judged in relation to its social origins; as well as implying potential, it also implies comparison.

Giftedness is often translated as high intelligence, even by some educational researchers who do not seem to have given the term proper scientific consideration. A baseline IQ point has historical precedent going back to Terman (1925) and also receives a degree of consensus. In the United States, researchers often take a baseline of IQ 130 (about 2% of the population) for the gifted, but in Britain, it is more often taken as IQ 140, i.e. about 0.4% of the population (Jensen, 1973b). Sometimes as much as the top 20% of children in IQ terms are called gifted. On the other hand, there are some educationalists who describe giftedness in personality or behaviour terms, such as non-conformity, exceptional perseverence, or extrasensory perception, whilst specific gifts, particularly of an artistic kind, are often called talents. A national investigation by Her Majesty's Inspectorate in Britain (DES, 1977) reported: 'The plain fact was that "giftedness" as a concept had not been thought about'. Headteachers in that survey seemed determined to see children as individuals and not to place them in any such category.

To be gifted is not just to have a very high IQ, but that helps. In the research described later (Chapter 4), I found that of parents who choose to describe their children as gifted in the North West of England, 97% said it was because of their very high intelligence. The other 3% said it was because of their children's musical ability; no other ability was

2

mentioned as the reason for a child being gifted. In the definitions of giftedness throughout the ages, intelligence is not all-embracing, but it is the crucial thread which runs throughout. Considerable information has been amassed about the origins and development of intelligence and, whatever intelligence tests measure, they do measure it reliably, which is why the definition of giftedness based on an IQ measurement is amenable to research and is so frequently used. But it is essential that the researcher define his terms at the beginning so that the rest of us can know what concept is being referred to as giftedness in the research.

The definition of giftedness used by Eric Ogilvie (1973) in his survey of facilities for gifted children in Britain epitomizes the difficulties of presenting a precise guide:

'The term "gifted" is used to indicate any child who is outstanding in either a general or specific ability, in a relatively broad or narrow field of endeavour... Where generally recognised tests exist as (say) in the case of "intelligence", then giftedness would be defined by test scores. Where no recognised tests exist it can be assumed that the subjective opinions of originality and imagination displayed would be the criteria we have in mind'.

This definition is open-ended and could not be called either rigorous or precise. In order to be workable, a definition must be reliable – i.e. giving the same results repeatedly, and valid – i.e. it should be true to the concept on which it is built.

# TRADITIONAL VIEWS OF GIFTED CHILDREN

Perhaps the most famous description of the gifted came from Plato. Over 2000 years ago, he described men of superior intellect as 'men of gold', as distinct from those of 'silver', 'iron' or 'brass'. Without further knowledge of his works, it might be thought that Plato was referring to the brightest and best of all mankind, but in fact he was not. He was, of course, a product of his time and although his thinking was advanced, if not scandalous for its day, he never did consider *all* children to have the same rights to education.

Plato's golden children would be boys who came from the Patrician class; he could only draw them from a select, tiny percentage of the population, while the rest would mostly not even learn to read. He advocated special education for these boys to increase their capacity for leadership, though many of them would have been given leadership irrespective of their gifts, because of their birth. Plato's golden children could be described in present day terms as gilded lilies.

Many hundreds of educational years later, Francis Galton's views on 'The Classification of Men' (1869) continued in a similar vein. He is arguing for evidence that men are not born equal in ability:

'There can hardly be surer evidence of the enormous difference between the intellectual capacity of men, than the prodigious differences in the numbers of marks obtained by those who gain mathematical honours at Cambridge'.

He recognizes that there are different kinds of students at Cambridge:

'the large bulk of Cambridge men are taken almost haphazard. A boy is intended for some profession . . . and is sent to Oxford or Cambridge'.

Galton's use of the word 'haphazard' has little to do with the present-day statistical term 'random sample'. These were the sons of the social elite of the country, which had been preselected for education over centuries on the basis of considerations other than ability. However, he says, there are:

'many others who have fairly won their way to the Universities and are therefore selected from an enormous area'.

Again his sample is far from random. It would be necessary to ask about the schools that the boys went to before they came to university, how they were permitted to become enrolled at that school and what sort of families they came from. In addition:

'Unfortunately for my purposes, the marks are not published. They are not even assigned on a uniform system, since each examiner is permitted to employ his own scale of marks'.

Nevertheless, in spite of not knowing who they were or how or why the students were at Cambridge, having no idea of their motivations, either to obtain high marks or kill time, and having no means of comparing the marks that were obtained, he concludes what he wanted to conclude. No doubt he is right – that some boys are better at getting higher marks in maths than others – but for all his undoubted genius, that conclusion is intelligent opinion and not scientific evidence.

Statistically, his case would not hold water for a moment. It is only quite recently, when social psychology has begun to emerge as a science, that an attempt began to be made to place the individual in the context of his social upbringing and life-chances. Retrospective studies of genius, such as that of Catharine M. Cox (1926), are subject to the same failure of understanding of social context. Cox set out to study the lives of people who had been great and famous. She wanted to see whether there were

4

any particular traits which these people showed as children and whether they could be identified as predictors of genius. She concluded that:

'Achievements like these are not the accidents of the day. They are the natural outgrowth in individuals of superior general powers of persistent interest and great zeal combined with rare talents'.

Again, this is undoubtedly true – for the individuals she studied; they were eminently brilliant and successful. But it does not allow us to make assumptions about the rest of the population, who were not only barred from most forms of education, but heavily sanctioned into their allotted places in life by the society of the time. It can be argued that there may have been others, showing quite different childhood traits, who were mentally and physically subdued into ignoring their abilities and accepting their lot. Had they received the same support as the more privileged, their contributions to life might have been very different.

There have been and still are geniuses in the world. These are people who make a significant change in the behaviour of nations or who reach the highest levels of achievement that humans, as distinct from gods, can attain (Roget, 1962). Genius has an unearthly, inexplicable quality and every genius is a unique individual. However, very few gifted children will ever grow up into that category, which is an extremely small one.

## THE MYTHOLOGY OF GIFTEDNESS

Social mythology is not dead. The old Greek and Roman stories which we recognize as myths are in fact only ancient ones; life is as steeped in mythology today as it always has been. Mythology is a way of perceiving the world – not imagination, which implies a contact with reality, but belief. The making and spreading of myths is the product of deep, illogical, emotional drives, emerging from a state of tension. A myth that some other and better way of life can or should exist is easier to believe in than the present, imperfect situation, whatever that is. Mythic thinking can become an acceptable, if distorted version of life, while logic is no answer to such belief which has its own reason for existence because it springs from emotion. Either logic or scientific evidence may disprove a myth, but it will not kill it.

The concept of the gifted child is particularly subject to long-held, customary attitudes and mythic thinking. In spite of well established research evidence to the contrary (Terman, 1925), gifted children are most often seen as physically underdeveloped and mentally distressed in a normal life situation. The opposite is scientifically true, but variations from this old myth of the unhappy gifted child are not always welcome or unacceptable. Virginia Woolf was aware of this when describing her half-sister, in a letter to her nephew (Woolf, 1978):

> 'she was often bewildered by the eccentric storms in which your grandfather indulged, ascribed by her too simply to the greatness of his intellect . . .'

The psychologist P.E. Vernon made the same point (Vernon *et al.*, 1977):

> 'The very bright child, according to traditional lore, is poorly developed physically, short sighted, no good at athletics; also precocity is flash-in-the-pan and doesn't last'.

The earlier a gifted child is identified, the more likely he is to adapt to the prescription, rather than the description. The identifier declares the tenets of mythology about gifted children to be true because he feels that they ought to be true and then behaves in ways that will make them true. For example, parents are in a particularly powerful position as identifiers. As parents, they have obviously exercised profound effects since the child was born and they will continue to be influential from identification onwards. Children identified as gifted may indeed be gifted, but that in itself cannot produce all the abnormal behaviour that is claimed for gifted children, such as that they are 'prone to sudden bursts of rage resulting from frustration' (Hopkinson, 1978). Some of the children's behaviour must be the direct result of the adult's belief that they are reacting to the stress of the mediocrity around them; for it is part of the mythology of gifted children that they should be so.

It is not difficult to imagine a family group imposing the mythic mantle of giftedness on to a bright child. Every sign of even normal ability is applauded as though it were exceptional and even indications of disturbance are welcomed for they add to the evidence that this is a gifted child who has the mythical difficulty of living in a mediocre world. Any piece of behaviour is interpretable in a wide variety of ways and it is not too difficult for parents to assimilate potentially discrepant evidence into an already existing mythic stereotype. These are judgements made within a social context; the final outcome is not dependent on the actions of a single child but of the other people involved. These others may be only strangers who provide an audience for the child's behaviour, but there are subtle social pressures affecting the behaviour of everyone involved and guiding them in a particular direction.

Sometimes, in seeking to interpret an apparently inexplicable argument, it is useful to turn it upside-down, and using this exercise with the myth of the gifted child is particularly informative. The myth expresses belief in the effect of stress bringing about 'deviance'. It may *not* be gifted children that need protection from the world because of their stressful situation and inherent weakness but the equally mythical power of the gifted which requires the world to be protected from them. Looking from an alternative perspective at the relationship between the gifted and their particular strength allows different interpretations of the efforts to make special provision for these children. In that sense, the emotion behind the myth may not be an altruistic desire for the good of gifted children, but fear of their potential power. The example below was described by Arthur Koestler (1976); although extreme, it makes a relevant point:

'Among the Volga Bulgars, Jon Fadlan found a strange custom: When they observe a man who excels through quickwittedness and knowledge, they say: "for this one it is more befitting to serve our Lord". They seize him, put a rope round his neck and hang him on a tree where he is left until he rots away . . .

Commenting on this passage, the Turkish orientalist Zeki Togan . . . has this to say: "There is nothing mysterious about the cruel treatment meted out by the Bulgars to people who were overly clever. It was based on the simple, sober reasoning of the average citizens who wanted to lead what they considered to be a normal life and to avoid any risk or adventure into which the 'genius' might lead them". He then quotes a Tartar proverb: "If you know too much, they will hang you, and if you are too modest, they will trample on you". He concludes that the victim "should not be regarded simply as a learned person but as an unruly genius, one who is too clever by half". This leads one to believe that the custom should be regarded as a measure of social defence against change, a punishment of non-conformists and potential innovators.'

A fear of normal children's power is common to all cultures. There are a wide variety of laws which prohibit children from exercising the power of decision over their own lives and especially the lives of others. Obvious examples are those of choice between parents when there is a divorce, or a genuine voice in the running of school affairs.

For the individual child, where he can adapt his behaviour to conform to adult standards, he will be seen as 'good' and consequently less subject to instruction. But where the adult type of behaviour which is expected of him is beyond the child's reach, such as with certain 'gifted' children, the expectation may generate frustration, feelings of

7

inadequacy and shame. Schools are structured to usher children through from their supposed time of inherent wilfulness and indiscipline into the calm of ordered mature life. They serve to orientate children to the social norms and ethics of the society around, so that the young might not discover for themselves 'incorrect' ways of behaving. In the case of gifted children, their potential for learning – and therefore also for deviant learning – is greater.

The influence of mythology in relation to gifted children can also be seen in the development of the English educational system. In mediaeval times, the few poor boys who were recognized as gifted were permitted a free but highly restricted education in grammar schools. However, there was later some feeling against this selection and intellectual channelling, as Winstanley, a 'leveller', wrote in 1652 (Hill, 1975):

'One sort of children shall not be trained up only to book learning and no other employment, called scholars, as they are in the government of monarchy; for then through idleness and exercised wit therein they spend their time to find out policies to advance themselves to be lords and masters above their labouring brethren.'

Later still, these schools tended to be taken over by the social elite and provided the basis for the public school system, for which entry was based on parental position. A new system of grammar schools was then created by local education authorities from the beginning of this century, catering mainly for middle class children, with the addition of some intellectually bright 'scholarship' recruits from lower down the social scale. After the Second World War, all British children were divided into bright and less than bright by a selective examination at the age of eleven-plus. The bright went to grammar schools, which still provided a fairly restricted academic education, while the rest of the child population were to be trained for lower level occupations. Recent government moves to make 'comprehensive' all secondary schools have brought about the cry that our educational standards will fall and that the gifted will be wasted. Perhaps the real fear is not so much that gifted children will be wasted, but that instead they will be free of the academic curriculum and turn their talents elsewhere. To a traditional academically tuned mind, the word 'wasted', when applied to a gifted child, means non-academic. Perhaps, instead of bewailing the fear of wastage among gifted children, it would be more truthful and less mythic to recognize the fear of the 'misuse' of power by future independently minded gifted adults.

A science fiction book, *The Midwich Cuckoos* (Wyndham, 1969), expresses this fear of gifted children most succinctly; briefly, an alien being places supremely gifted children into an English village. The knowingness, inexplicability and mental superiority of the children is the source of fear, which in the story is found to be warranted when it is discovered that they are in fact the product of a higher power, which is about to take over the world. As with Koestler's example, these much too gifted children are disposed of in the end, though this was certainly not seen as waste, for both their power and the reader's fear were explicit. The myth was exposed here to strong dramatic effect, but because myth is based on emotion perhaps it is only in a form of expression such as drama, or through sophisticated psychological analysis, that its reality will ever be fully understood.

Genius has often been thought of as akin to madness, but this axiom has little evidence to support it. In fact, the occasional genius who becomes mentally disturbed has often had his creativity curtailed, for instance, Nijinsky or Virginia Woolf. Other highly gifted creators, such as Van Gogh and Edward Munch, showed evidence of psychiatric abnormalities in the increasingly strange quality of their paintings, but when the severity of the mental illness became too great, they too had their creative processes destroyed. The conclusion of the French sociologist Foucault is probably a just one: 'Madness is an absolute break with the world of art' (quoted by Wing, 1978).

However, the lesser association between giftedness and eccentricity has probably been of help to people over the centuries. The Court Fool, for example, was also a 'wise man', the only one of his Court who could speak to the King directly and honestly. Shakespeare illustrated this by putting social criticism into the mouths of 'fools'. Eccentric behaviour can still be an acceptable cover for insights and wisdom, where these are not seen as being socially appropriate, while some of the contemporary 'lunatic fringe' – people who act well beyond the bounds of convention – may not be lunatic at all, but too clever by half.

## THE MEDICAL MODEL OF ABNORMALITY

The development of psychology has paralleled, if slowly, the development of scientific medicine. For centuries, explanations of behaviour which was considered to be odd were offered in terms of belief in interfering superior forces; they also reflected deep social attitudes as to what was acceptable behaviour for that particular group of people.

What was health and what was not health depended for definition on a wide variety of clues. For example, it might be difficult to tell if a person showing evidence of disturbance was suitable to be treated by doctors or by someone who had command over unseen powers.

As medicine became more scientific, certain patterns of behaviour began to become definable in terms of specific theories which are testable. Rather than assigning puzzling conditions to the realm of magic, there began to be systematic research into their origins and treatment; for medicine, this was the recognition of disease. But whether these patterns of behaviour were regarded as in need of alteration depended to a large extent on what was regarded as socially undesirable. The old ways are with us still, even though the received attitude is that of science. Writing on the medical model, John Wing, the social psychiatrist, says (Wing, 1978):

> 'Because few societies are likely to regard musical or mathematical genius as undesirable it is most improbable (though not impossible) that either will ever be called a disease'

Disease is regarded as a deviant and distinctive pattern of behaviour with clusters of specific syndromes that are susceptible to treatment. Being gifted, as described by many educationalists, comes into this category of disease, although the word 'disease' itself is never used.

The process of selection of gifted children in itself assumes the existence of a distinctive and measurable pattern of behaviour. As with any other diagnosis, the selection of children as gifted presupposes some related form of treatment or education. But the identification of gifted children has by no means yet been perfected. Previously satisfactory ability tests are not always acceptable now, as they are deemed to discriminate against deprived groups, such as those of low socio-economic status or ethnic minorities. Suggested methods of identification are often behavioural, for instance (Lyon, 1976):

> 'These are the youngsters who ask the "threatening" questions in the classroom'

The implication is that they bring out hostility in teachers and thus teachers' supposed ill-feelings towards them are understandable. Again (The Daily Telegraph (London), May 29, 1974):

> 'Highly gifted children are in danger of becoming drop-outs and delinquents, or even super-cunning criminals, because schools are failing to give them an education that matches their abilities, head teachers said yesterday.'

*10*

Medical treatment can be as odd as the description of the symptoms, e.g. in *The Life of Noel Coward,* an undoubtedly gifted child (Lesley, 1976):

> 'When Noel was still two the doctor pronounced that his brain was much in advance of his body and advised that he should be left very quiet, that all his curls should be cut off and that he was to go to no parties.'

Working to well defined behavioural descriptions of giftedness, educationalists and psychologists can devise methods of education which will undoubtedly be beneficial. That is, the symptoms may become fewer or less objectionable and the child happier. But because we do not really know the root causes of these problems, there can be no generally applicable education for gifted children. We remain unsure quite how much of the benefit is due to the increased attention or to the specific child-centred education which is being provided, or how much any normal child would benefit by such a tailor-made programme.

As with disease or any other 'abnormality', it would be foolish to provide treatment or education especially designed for that condition, while ignoring the wider psychological and social context. That would be as if, in deciding on a course of treatment, the designer were wearing a pair of psychological blinkers and naturally this would make vision very circumscribed. The practice of treating gifted children with special educational programmes, regardless of the rest of the educational situation, e.g. by isolating them in special schools, calls for a considerable narrowness of view. Whatever the outcomes of such a situation, they can only be considered in relation to the experience of children of all abilities in other situations. Schooling in a social vacuum is not education and it is a matter of concern when administrators behave or want to behave as if it could be carried out that way. Such policies may have little to do with reason or logic and much to do with ingrained social attitudes. Again, as with medicine, the larger the social influence on diagnosis, the less likely is it that the diagnosis will be accurate.

There is a side-effect of the medical model, which is that of the 'sick-role', and children, especially bright ones, are not slow to take up the special privileges and position of the 'sick'. These may lead over time to the accentuation of extra personal and social handicaps, which are really nothing to do with being gifted. Rather, they are a direct product of the process of being diagnosed, labelled and categorized as 'gifted' and thus in need of special treatment. Such sick-role behaviour may not develop at all, should the reaction of adults – and possibly educational policy – be different. Being gifted may be seen as a considerable social handicap, where no handicap need have existed before, and so may become one. I have heard more than one parent say 'he can't possibly get on with other children; he's so gifted that they can't understand him' or 'he's too sensitive to play with other children who are not of his kind'.

When children, or adults for that matter, are out of step with what is considered to be normal, they ask for advice from someone who is deemed to have superior knowledge. Children who have a sore throat are seen by a medical doctor; children who are believed to be gifted are seen by a psychologist or a teacher. It is important to recognize that the adults involved in bringing the child to notice are very often concerned about her outward behaviour and not necessarily her abilities. In addition, it depends on the psychologist's own beliefs whether she says 'the child is gifted; therefore you must expect this behaviour' or simply 'your child has scored high (or low) on the test, but her behaviour problems need attention'. In their recommendations, psychologists and teachers are affected by social norms, over and above their professional skills; it is well-nigh impossible to be an objective judge of another's behaviour when one is a member of the same social system. Sometimes the label of gifted will be offered merely as a reassurance to worried parents, or to fit in with the filing system. Such diagnoses do not necessarily depend on an understanding of causation, nor are they always made with a view to prescribing treatment. The diagnostic identification can be an end in itself, carrying implications of disturbance which are unavoidable.

In fact, the medical model is often used unrecognized in the identification of gifted children. In the United States, for example, many local education authorities issue check-lists of normal behaviour, by which teachers can begin to sift out their pupils for special treatment. Writers of books for parents and teachers often provide these lists, as do organizations for the gifted. It is my belief that the production of such lists and the descriptions of gifted children mentioned above require a much closer look in respect of their social origins.

The diagnosis or labelling of a child as gifted implies a whole dynamic set of associated ideas and assumptions, derived as much from myth and wishful thinking as from scientific evidence. But there is actually so little relevant scientific evidence that its representation in diagnosis (or identification) must be small. The medical model has enabled psychology to find its scientific feet, but its thrusting expansionism must be held in check. It does not always have an adequate goodness of fit and the present discussion of giftedness is one example of this. But it is available to be tested and must be modified or rejected, to the extent that it fails any relevant tests; if it passes them, we must assume that yet further tests lie ahead. A scientist asks simply that before being accepted all theories should receive the same treatment and should be able to stand up to scrutiny.

Unfortunately, the scientific approach is not amenable to historical insight, nor does it allow for the development and handing down of a tradition of caring, based on experience, intuition and interaction with children. But in order for it to be scientific, there is no need to throw out these invaluable assets along with the unwarranted assumptions.

## IDENTIFYING GIFTED CHILDREN

Even before we can begin to consider the problems of identification of gifted children, those of general recognition have to be looked at first. It cannot be taken for granted that the gifted child is recognized as a special category of child at all, much less that such a child must have problems. It can be argued that what some may consider to be the problems of giftedness are so insignificant, if not illusory, that they are not worthy of either consideration or action. In addition, since these so-called problems are not as obvious as, for instance, those of mongolism, they are sometimes said to be not worth searching out.

Headteachers in Britain are not, on the whole, in favour of recognizing giftedness as a problem. They see the National Association for Gifted Children (UK) as a middle-class pressure group, fighting for special recognition of the gifted child, who has a low priority as far as they are concerned. In fact, when I asked some headteachers for permission to conduct research on the subject in their schools, the request was occasionally seen as a form of middle-class, academic interference. As such, it was to be stamped on at the outset. Teachers in some schools see the term gifted as synonymous with demanding parents and difficult children; when a child bears the label of gifted in that type of school, it will not be to his advantage. Where the problems of giftedness are recognized as existing, it is usual for a teacher to see those problems in terms of the individual child, rather than as a category of all gifted children (Ogilvie, 1973: DES, 1977). Perhaps in the present state of confusion and lack of evidence, this is the safest, if not the most constructive approach.

But in spite of the barriers of entrenched attitudes, progress has certainly been made in identifying gifted children. Much of this work, though, has been done in the United States and unfortunately is not always relevant to the British educational system or way of life. Since all identification is a matter of description and classification, it can only be effective in terms of comparison. Thus a child is gifted amongst other children and not by itself. In general, we are still very largely in the observational stage in respect of giftedness and it will be a matter of time for these methods of identification to be further tested and improved.

But when a gifted child is identified now, some pertinent questions should be asked. Does the identification help the individual and if so how? Does it enable predictions to be made about the child's future? Will this identification help others? Are families helped by being offered a socially acceptable label to their problem? How has it come about that this child is receiving extra attention? Giftedness may be identified in terms of specific abilities or as an all-round bundle' of potential, but from either point of view, the events preceding identification and definition are obviously crucial if further action is to be based on it.

Although we can now recognize descriptive signs of giftedness, we still need more assurance of their validity. A further requirement is a knowledge of which of these discriminating signs are accompanied by others, which are not in themselves discriminating. Thus, a high IQ may in itself be a discriminatory and even measurable sign, but we cannot say for certain whether this gift is accompanied by any linked behaviour. My research (described later in Chapter 4) has shown that a high IQ of itself does not cause difficult behaviour in children. But this evidence is the first of its kind and would benefit from similar, cross-cultural studies. There is also the problem of specific gifts, which appear to come in pairs or groups. For example, mathematics and music are commonly considered, even by specialist teachers in these subjects, to come together. In fact, while there is no evidence to merit this assumption, there has been evidence against it; in her study of the inheritance of musical ability, Shuter (1968) found that music is largely a singular, specific gift. She concluded that any connection that musical talent might have with mathematical/scientific ability was due to an all-round 'integrated intellect', but could not otherwise be accepted as an established pairing. Revesz (1953) found that only 9% of professional musicians had mathematical talent or interest in mathematics. Unfortunately, the large investigation at Johns Hopkins University (Stanley, Keating and Fox, 1974) on mathematically gifted children did not investigate the possibility of a musical link.

A favourite method of recognizing and identifying gifted children is to draw up a list of their 'characteristics'. The lists begin with a small selection of characteristics, such as intense curiosity, independence of mind or early reading, but there are always children who are exceptions to each. A particular child does not always fit exactly, so that the lists grow to accommodate the exceptions and as they grow longer and more impressive over the passage of time, they also become more all-embracing until some of them would describe almost any child. To say, for example, that a characteristic of a gifted child is that she asks a lot of questions tells us little, because children brought up in an atmosphere which encourages such behaviour will do so. There are equally gifted children who do not ask many questions because it is disapproved of and so they take pains to control the flow. Other characteristics and abilities may also be concealed if children find them unacceptable to people they value; these people may be adults or other children. Fashion, too is important; the primary characteristic described for a socially gifted child in America in the 1950s was general physical attractiveness with neatness in appearance – perhaps this fashion will return some day.

The makers of some lists suggest that if you can tick a certain proportion of characteristics with regard to your child, then you have identified him as gifted. But what most listmakers actually say is that there are some characteristics frequently found in gifted children and they hope only to stimulate a parent or teacher's suspicions that a child might be gifted. The next move would be to approach an 'authority' on the subject. However, the lists themselves really fail as identification tools because they have no predictive or definitive value. The following list from the Department of Education and Science (UK) (Hoyle and Wilks, 1975) is typical:

### Gifted children: A teacher's checklist

Exceptionally able children are likely to show the following characteristics.

A child showing most characteristics on the checklist, but not those starred, is likely to be a gifted child who is under-achieving educationally.

1. Possess superior powers of reasoning, of dealing with abstractions, of generalizing from specific facts, of understanding meanings, and of seeing into relationships.

2. Have great intellectual curiosity.

3. Learn easily and readily.

4. Have a wide range of interests

5. Have a broad attention-span that enables them to concentrate on, and persevere in solving problems and pursuing interests.

6. Are superior in the quantity and quality of vocabulary as compared with the children of their own age.

7. Have ability to do effective work independently.

8. Have learned to read early (often well before school age).

9. Exhibit keen powers of observation.

10. Show initiative and originality in intellectual work.

11. Show alertness and quick response to new ideas.

12. Are able to memorize quickly.

13. Have great interest in the nature of man and the universe (problems of origins and destiny, etc.).

14. Possess unusual imagination.

15. Follow complex directions easily.

16. Are rapid readers.

17. Have several hobbies.

18. Have reading interests which cover a wide range of subjects.

19. Make frequent and effective use of the library.

20. Are superior in mathematics, particularly in problem solving.

Lists are probably unavoidable in helping towards the identification of any condition, but some are less emotionally loaded and more helpful than others. The list which follows (Ward, 1975) is described as being centred upon 'the most clearly known deviant characteristics, i.e.: general intellectual superiority'. It is intended to be helpful to educators, particularly for screening and identification. Certainly it is comprehensive and accurate, but its practical use is as yet nebulous. The intellectual characteristics described are mostly those picked up by intelligence tests, which are in fact practical, reliable and excellent predictors of scholastic achievement.

*Capacity for Learning:* Accurate perception of social and natural situations; independent, rapid, efficient learning of fact and principle; fast, meaningful reading, with superior retention and recall.

*Power and Sensitivity of Thought:* Ready grasp of principles underlying things as they are; sensitivity to interference in fact, consequence of proposition, application of idea; spontaneous elevation of immediate observations to higher planes of abstraction; imagination; meaningful association of ideas; forceful reasoning; original interpretations and conclusions; discriminatory power, quick detection of similarities and differences among things and ideas; able in analysis, synthesis, and organization of elements, critical of situations, self, and other people.

*Curiosity and Drive:* Mental endurance; tenacity of purpose; stubbornness, sometimes contrarily expressed as reluctance to do as directed; capacity for follow-through with extensive, but meaningful plans; curiosity about things and ideas; intrinsic interest in the challenging and difficult; versatile and vital interests; varied, numerous and penetrating inquiries; boredom with routine and sameness.

The distinction between potential and achievement relative to other children is vitally important in identifying giftedness. The child whose home background has enabled her to exercise her abilities and to achieve highly is more likely to be identified as gifted than the one from a restricted home. This is a considerable problem, especially in a school serving a poor community, where there is a tendency for teachers to lose heart over their unprepossessing charges. I have myself heard teachers say that there are no gifted children in their schools as they are 'only council children', meaning that they live in city council subsidized housing.

## PRESENT INTEREST IN GIFTED CHILDREN

To be interested in gifted children must involve distinguishing between children as a whole. Some call this an 'elitist' way of thinking in the sense that it implies priority for a part of the population. But to say that all children are of equal ability is to deny the overwhelming evidence to the contrary. As interest in gifted children has grown considerably in the last decade and has been given approval and recognition by various governments, it is pertinent to ask why this is so, as it is most certainly related to the socal issues of our time. The study of gifted children in their social contexts, described in Chapter 4 of this book, was concerned with identifying some of the prevailing attitudes and expectations of parents and teachers about this subject.

*17*

Theorizing without respect for the test of facts and collecting data without using them to test theory are not in any terms scientific. Yet much of the information which circulates about gifted children is written by people who 'know from experience' and who thus regard themselves as able to present their opinions as facts. Such 'information' is generally accepted because of the lack of data obtained from scientific research on what is involved in being described as 'gifted'.

The subject of giftedness attracts both prophets and politicians, most of whom are not concerned in any way with testing their proposals; they only want to be believed. Such people are most frequently heard or seen on the media, but there are others, more subtle opinionizers, who are capable of reinterpreting information and who appear to be offering a scientifically based set of facts from which they have drawn their conclusions. In fact, they are presenting no more than their own individual vision, which has the validity of a work of imagination rather than of one of science. In the end, the theory which is accepted is not necessarily the one which has passed the most stringent scientific experiments; it is the one which corresponds best with the social myth of the time. The scientific approach does not vary, no matter what is being investigated, but the initial theory and plan of investigation is directly attributable to prevailing social circumstances and to the beliefs and attitudes of the people involved. These will also affect the conclusions drawn from the results. Durkheim in his work on suicide first showed that behaviour has a social reference, that it is both individual *and* social (Durkheim, 1952). He showed that suicide was not only the behaviour of an individual, but that it was more likely to occur in certain social situations than others. Before Durkheim, the prevailing theory had been the 'historicist' view, meaning that history would repeat itself, given the same circumstances. But in fact, circumstances are never identical; the world (or society) is dynamic and we who live in it must live in our own time. It follows that we have to examine our world from the point of view of the present era and not as it was or how we would like it to be.

Interest in gifted children has varied around the world with the value placed on children's abilities. When cheap clerical labour was considered to be valuable in Victorian England, intellectually gifted boys were appraised and trained for that narrow role in elementary schools. Pasold (1977), an industrialist, describes such a person:

'. . . it seems incredible that Mr. Colmer, our Chief Clerk, kept the books, recorded movements of stocks of raw material and finished goods, did the costings and prepared the weekly profit or loss statements all in ink and in longhand. He hardly ever made a mistake. He also calculated and paid the wages.'

Today, a political interest in gifted children is again focussed on their economic value and in a world of shrinking resources we need their gifts to enable civilisation, as the West knows it, to continue. Gifted children could provide endless natural power, if only we knew how to harness it.

Individuals become interested in gifted children for many reasons. Some feel that this is a part of the child population which is not receiving an education appropriate to their abilities; in that sense, gifted children are deprived. Carrying this idea further, highly gifted children have recently been called 'severely' gifted, the implications being of handicap. This emotive labelling is presumably designed to draw attention to the plight of the gifted in the educational system. The deprived minority of gifted children thus provides an acceptable political platform and it is currently more fashionable to demand help for a minority group than better education for all. It also provides new fields of venture and employment for academics and educationalists.

Identification with the gifted child may also provide adults with consolation for their own lost childhoods. In caring for gifted children, they may remember what it was like to be a gifted child in a world where no-one understood, or may make-believe that they themselves would have been gifted if only things had been different.

Worldwide, the general interest in gifted children is steadily gathering momentum; societies exist on behalf of them and government departments set aside money for research and help for their education. The World Council for Gifted Children was formed in 1975 and has already held two international congresses, while in America, the National Merit Scholarship Program stands as evidence of a national commitment to identify and support intellectual excellence. Although interest in giftedness is often said to be in respect of all abilities, intellectual or mathematical abilities command the lion's share of attention in the developed, technological world. This is in fact what would be expected in view of the determination of the concept of giftedness by social and cultural forces, which has been described in this chapter.

# CHAPTER 2

# Learning to be Gifted

It is certain that learning begins before birth. From about four months after conception, a foetus can be observed at various stages of its development to be undergoing learning processes; sounds, movements and pressures inside the uterus constitute its environment. Even at this period, the baby has innate reflexes which can be used for learning and which can be seen when babies who have been born before full term respond to bright light or startling noise. A baby's learning in response to the behaviour of others is social learning and there are a number of theories as to the processes by which it takes place.

It is primarily society, in the form of other people, which acts on the infant to mould its behaviour by socialization. But clearly, since the same social environmental conditions produce different reactions in different children, the infant cannot be merely a passive recipient of fortune's handouts. His own developing knowingness (cognition) is considered to act as mediator between himself and the outside world. In this personal way, he contributes to his own social development. The psychologist's problem is to understand the relative interactive effects of these two social forces – other people and the child himself – in an individual's social learning.

The aspects of social learning which are discussed in this chapter are those which are particularly relevant to gifted children. They are presented successively in terms of the individual, the small group of which he is a part and the society and culture which encompasses them all.

# THE INDIVIDUAL

The nature–nurture controversy has been raging for centuries and evidence continues to pile up on both sides. Professor Higgins in Shaw's *Pygmalion* sided entirely with the nurture camp when he effectively re-made the flower-girl into a duchess. Watson, in the early part of the century, committed himself wholeheartedly in the same direction (Watson, 1925):

> 'Give me a dozen healthy infants, well formed and my own specified world to bring them up in and I'll guarantee to take any one at random and train him to become any kind of specialist I might select – doctor, lawyer, beggarman and thief, regardless of his talents, penchants, tendencies, abilities, vocation and race of his ancestors'.

Watson is often called the father of *behaviourism*; he believed we can alter children's behaviour at will by changing their environment. He aimed to construct a set of universal laws applicable to all human behaviour, but even in the animal world, it has long been seen how different species have adapted their behaviour to fit in with their environments.

B.F. Skinner (1953), also a committed behaviourist, actually put theory into practice; not having a dozen healthy infants to work with, he chose his second daughter. As a baby, she spent long hours in his 'air crib' – a large sound-proofed and air-conditioned box. She was then in a comfortable, germ-free atmosphere, which made blankets or clothing unnecessary. She could view the outside world from it and be put in and taken out for feeding and cuddling via a glass window. In replying to the furore of criticism which this action produced, Skinner replied that it was only the 'artificiality' of the situation which was raising hackles. He saw his daughter's environment as a simple, comfortable one that had been mechanically devised for a specific purpose. She has grown up, as far as we know, to be healthy, happy – and highly intelligent.

Contrary to the old behaviourist view that environment is almost wholly responsible for developing behaviour, the geneticists place their faith in the inheritance of abilities. Although there is argument about the exact proportions, many present-day genetic psychologists have concluded from research results that only 20% of a child's behaviour is affected by environmental circumstances; the other 80% has been effectively determined at conception. The logical consequences of this standpoint would be to put less effort into improving a child's learning enviroment, to accept children as they come and, instead of trying to 'improve' them, to allow them to develop in their own ways.

Psychologists such as Eysenck and Jensen accept this view that the possibility of individual change is limited to such an extent. Jencks (1973) suggested that schools have very little effect and that society could be 'deschooled' with little detriment to anyone. From the geneticist's perspective, gifted children are born and not made. Since by this reasoning they are very few in number, their precious potential warrants skilled nurturing. When educational resources are limited (as they nearly always are), education should therefore be given as appropriate to the child and not as a universal right of ever-open choice. The decision as to how to educate any child would then have to be based on some kind of measurement. In fact, this viewpoint did effectively change the face of British education for many years. Under the guidance of Burt, the genetic psychologist, children were selected for their education by virtue of their ability, as measured by tests constructed for that purpose.

However, most working psychologists do not take such extreme positions, but pick and choose from theory and practice; that is, they have an eclectic approach. It is assumed in this book that some unknown proportion of ability is inherited. But we do not even know if the inheritance of ability is in identical proportions for each individual; abilities are flexible and subject to many influences, as this chapter describes.

My concern has been to investigate, both theoretically and practically, environmental influences on the development of children's abilities. Circumstances affect children of very high ability, as well as the less able, but we have almost no evidence as to how, or in what way, such influences may be different for gifted children. The distinction between the recognition of giftedness in a child by others and the child's own growing awareness of his gifts is confused, but open to exploration. Although it is only behaviour that is actually observable, an understanding of the events leading up to it, and the ways in which it may be measured, serve to place it in perspective.

## Conditioning

In 1927, the Russian psychologist Pavlov carried out a series of experiments on dogs to discover how and when they salivated in response to food. He discovered that a reflex response (salivation) could be brought about by bringing food near to the dog. Later, it was found that if he rang a bell at the same time as he brought the food, the same reflex response happened. The next experimental move was to ring only the bell; he found that a dog that was used to the bell and food together still gave the salivation response. Pavlov called this a *conditioned reflex,* the bell was the conditional stimulus for the reflex. He also discovered that the dog would not salivate to the bell alone for long; it had to have more *reinforcement,* i.e. more food. A dog could also *generalize*; hearing different bells produced the same conditioned reflex. Humans too often react to various stimuli with reflexes, whether unconditional like the knee-jerk, or conditional like mouth-watering at the smell of food. It is conceivable that we have chains of reflexes, varying from the simple eye-blink to thoughts of pure philosophy, all based on the basic principle that Pavlov discovered.

Operant conditioning, which B.F. Skinner (1953) has worked on for many years, is a more complicated process. It is not dependent on a simple physical response, but is a product of the environment in which it occurs. Skinner pointed to the difference between Pavlov's simple stimulus–response reflexes, which he called *respondents,* and reflexes which happen without a known stimulus, called *operants.* It is operant behaviour which involves a child as a whole in relation to his environment, i.e. what he has to do in order to get his reward, or reinforcement.

Skinner describes his reinforcers as *positive* because there is an effort involved to get them; when an effort is made to avoid a situation, the reinforcement is termed *negative.* These operant reinforcers are therefore described by what they do. Any increase in the rate of reinforced behaviour is effective operant conditioning and it can be used to promote any type of behaviour.

Through operant conditioning, complex schedules of learning and reinforcement can be used to 'shape' behaviour. This is done by reinforcing any tendency in the required direction. Gradually, the criterion for presenting the reinforcer is shifted to be closer and closer to the targeted response until it occurs sufficiently often to merit direct reinforcement. In the everyday world, the reinforcer need only be a token like academic honours, money or medals. Token reinforcers are useless in themselves, but can be exchanged for other, more tangible things.

Adults have always used a form of operant conditioning to shape children's behaviour. Their positive reinforcers are for example, attention, approval or affection; negative reinforcers are anger, violence or withdrawn affection. They are not always given obviously and there are many subtle ways in which adults give reinforcement to children. For example, a girl may be 'allowed' to overhear herself being praised for getting good marks at school, or a boy may hear his mother describing his aggressive behaviour and referring to him as 'a real boy'.

However, children can be mistaken in their interpretations of adult messages since their knowledge and perspectives are limited by their experience. Messages are often confused, either in delivery or intention, which is disturbing to children. A gifted child may be both praised by his teacher for being top of the class, yet dismissed as a 'know-all' during lesson time. Parents who constantly complain about the trouble that their daughter's giftedness causes them, while at the same time leaving the impression of reflected glory, place her in an impossible position. She cannot please by being gifted, yet she will fail them if she is not gifted. Her lack of positive reinforcement and the presence of the negative reinforcement is a disturbing cocktail.

Theories of conditioning are limited by their dependence on what is observable and measurable. Although they provide an entirely practical emphasis, it is at the expense of a wide range of subtler subject matter which is neglected. Skinner is particularly concerned with the rate of behaviour, rather than its meaning to the individual. His disregard of the internal causes of behaviour and view of a total dependence on environmental conditions represent a one-sided limitation within the wide possibilities that psychology provides for understanding human activities. In brief, the frame of reference for conditioning is very restricted, but it is a usable and useful intellectual base from which behaviour can be manipulated, if not fully understood.

## Modelling

The American psychologist Bandura (1969) argued that conditioning theories would be too slow to account for all of a child's rapid social development. He sees social learning as being guided essentially by example. As part of the process of socialization, a child acquires behaviour by imitating that which first exists in another person – the exhibition of the action to him is sufficient for the child to incorporate it as his own. Bandura regards this theory as inadequate because in it the child has an entirely passive position. In his own concept of modelling, the external behaviour is not absorbed into the child in a pure form because the child cognitively acts on it, selecting from it and transforming it in the process of incorporation. In this way, there is a direct relationship between the other person's behaviour and the child's, but they are not exactly the same.

Where the child is seen as the passive recipient of social learning, he must be dependent for his social functioning on others. This direct influence would enable him to interact with other people and in these terms, as children develop, they would become more and more like the adults around them. But if the child's growing cognition (knowingness) acts as a mediator between him and the outside world, it would bring about an interpersonal correspondence between them – a shared understanding and shared, rather than copied, behaviour.

But, as a model, adult behaviour can be as confusing to follow as any other unclear message, with the same distressing results to the child. No matter how competent their mediation processes, children are often presented with a set of instructions which differ from the adult behaviour shown – 'Don't do as I do; do as I say'. Outside the family circle, there are other important models which do not have to be experienced at first hand to be effective. In Bandura's words (1967):

> 'film-mediated models are as effective as real-life models in eliciting and transmitting aggressive responses and can no longer be ignored in concep-tualisations of personality development. Indeed most youngsters probably have more exposure to male models than to their own fathers. With further advances in mass media and audio-visual technology, models presented pictorially, mainly through television, are likely to play an increasingly influential role in shaping personality patterns and in modifying attitudes and social norms.'

Should these findings be accepted by the media, they would obviously have profound effects on all forms of information processing. But for the time being, commercial entertainment and psychological knowledge are uncoordinated.

There is considerable agreement among contemporary psychologists that social learning does in fact take place via the child's cognitive mediation. During the process of incorporating other people's behaviour patterns within himself, the child's cognition acts to convert the pattern into some mental state. From there, it can be interpreted and used as the basis for the child's own behaviour. Gifted children may have more facility with cognitive mediation than other children. If so, this would give them a more flexible means of interpretation and behaviour and would enable them to act more independently than other children. A superior cognitive facility would be expected to provide the means by

*26*

which a child would be more aware and thus more sensitive to people and situations.

The intervention of cognition in the processes of social learning is difficult to disentangle. It serves at one and the same time as a mediator, the result of social learning and the basis by which the child might develop. It is a tool for grasping social knowledge – validly, mistakenly or not at all.

## Social interaction

Social learning can also be understood in terms of relationships between children and others. There are a number of theories of social development by interaction which have an overlapping consensus of argument, viz. social learning develops when children are with others in any form of relationship; the ever-changing end-product, social knowledge, is itself a relationship; social knowledge is based on an evolving system of mutually understood rules for interaction.

Children arrive at understandings between themselves and others in terms of how each is permitted to behave. All the people concerned in the interaction must have some shared comprehension of the appropriate structure for behaviour. Although adults have the upper hand in their relationships with children, by learning from these relationships children are able to relate more easily and quickly with strangers. Just a few experimental reactions will enable a new relationship to be made, based on old experiences.

It is from the idea that interaction takes place in a structure of mutually understood rules that deviance can be seen in terms of rule-breaking. What is seen as deviance depends on the perspective and tolerance of the viewer; an action that is deviant to you is not deviant to me. Gifted children are likely to be more independent of adult rule structures than other children. Consequently, they are more likely to be seen as 'difficult' and different, if not actually deviant. Children who conform to adult rules are seen as 'good', while independent thinking by children is confusing to adult expectations and threatening to their authority. The less stable the parents, the less able they will be to cope with irregular behaviour in their child. In order to be socially acceptable, gifted children are obliged to balance a fine tightrope between adult expectation and their own surges of independent thinking.

# THE GROUP

In a complex society, the social learning of an individual happens in the first place within the particular sub-culture or group in which the child is born. However the different organizations operating in society may have conflicting wishes and aims so that the balance of power and influence shifts between them. This power can be stable at times and at other times quite unstable, while the effects of the system's relative degree of stability are highly significant for the lives of the individuals involved. Greater societal instability strongly affects the various small groups of people that exist in it and can even cause them to break up as entities. Though social change is constant, its speed may vary from the barely perceivable to revolution.

A child is a member of several social groups of different sizes; as well as her family, they may be those of social class, religion, geographical area, sex or ethnic group. Social learning in groups is concerned with acquiring the specific patterns of behaviour which are suitable for those who are members of a group at any one time. In addition, it means learning the patterns of behaviour of members of this group in relation to other members of society.

## Socialization processes

Socialization is concerned with changes in attitudes and behaviour; it occurs through learning and particularly through interaction with others. An excellent explanation of socialization was given by Irwin Child (1954):

> 'Socialization is the process by which an individual born with behaviour potentialities of an enormously wide range is led to develop actual behaviour confined within the narrow range of what is customary for him according to the standards of the group.'

A child learns how to behave in the context of the other people, i.e. society; the unfolding genetic blueprint cannot ever proceed without some form of social interference. Socialization is in part conditioning and in part the interaction between inherited characteristics and circumstances. It is by this means that human babies grow up and adjust to their societies, so that they can continue living within them. Where socialization is not sufficiently accomplished, the individual may feel discomfort at being with other people, or may find it difficult or even impossible to fit in socially.

When social psychology was in its infancy, at the beginning of the twentieth century, it seemed to the early theorists that socialization was a method of slotting people into ways of life. It was as though the networks or organizations were kept going by the appropriate development of individuals to fit the system. In this way, the system and the individual fitted together and so society on the whole remained stable and did not change violently.

Since then, though, further evidence and thinking have clarified the situation. Western society is no longer regarded as a cultural unity; it has no collective mind and cannot tell people how to fit to its parameters. Few modern societies, in fact, are so overwhelmingly stable that they can direct the individuals within them to fulfil allotted functions throughout their lives. Most are complex and changing, so that there are diverse sub-cultures and groupings within the body of each society. These different parts may have conflicting aims, organizations, shifts of power and overlapping functions. Any one individual may travel through many such parts during a lifetime, though it is impossible fully to comprehend even all those with which a single person may come into contact.

## Roles

In its most frequently used sense, a role is that which an actor plays in his relationships with others on the stage, his own past forming one part of the plot. Social roles are not different in performance, but they are entirely different in the reality of the situation. A social role is not a fantasy or a pretence; for example, a mothering role must have a child or a child substitute, which can be mothered. It also has continuity of action since a single act does not in itself establish a role; that only grows out of familiarity and expectation. Other people then begin to act reciprocally and each can become an extension of the original role – a 'role other'. The pattern of role playing within a relationship works out to embrace action, acceptance and reciprocal action.

Individuals, caught in situations which are not of their choosing, can find themselves playing roles that are grindingly unsympathetic to them. A child can be forced into a role which is so far from his nature as to lead to misery, but the more adaptable a child is, the more he is able to manoeuvre himself into a modified role, which is easier for him to live with. A bright child, forced into playing the stereotyped role of 'gifted child', may be very distressed – and show it in his behaviour – or may modify his performance to that of an average child, thereby disappointing others but achieving a more tolerable existence for himself.

The 'gifted child'* has the problem of success incorporated into her role; she cannot walk away from failure. She has no choice and must go on being clever, even when it is not really possible for her to be so. Consequently, some 'gifted children' in fact live a life of constant failure in certain areas, or see themselves as living disappointments, having to act out their inability to achieve what others expect of them over and over again. In addition to primary 'failure' from insufficient achievement, secondary failure may result from the role of 'gifted child' being so diffuse that no child can fulfil it.

Role playing is a device for learning, but where it is based on falsehood and thus fails to communicate anything meaningful, it loses its usefulness. When young people are placed into stereotypes, i.e. inappropriate roles, they often recognize and resent the false, hurtful information that flows into them from that situation. This may cause the individual not only to modify the role, but to rebel against it or even to opt out of that part of the society which brought the situation about. Gifted children may slide into disruption because they cannot trust either their roles or their own identity, which drives them to such a state of distrust. But if the role has a real hold, the child cannot act outside the structure of that role; she is trapped.

Role changing and role breaking make heavy emotional demands on the player, as well as on the others who form part of the relationship which shaped that role. This is particularly so when the reason for role change is disillusionment; children can then suffer permanent emotional scarring. The breakdown in role can be very frightening to those involved and dealing with the resulting emotions of anger and hostility may need skilled professional help.

## Sex-differences in roles

It may seem that to sub-divide the role of gifted child by sex is splitting hairs, but there are very notable differences in the behaviour of parents towards their gifted boys and girls respectively.

The most striking fact about the children whose parents believed them to be gifted in my research was that twice as many parents of boys had joined the National Association for Gifted Children as parents of girls. Also, in proportion to their numbers, twice as many boys (70%) as girls (35%) were seen by their parents and their teachers as being

---

* 'gifted child' in inverted commas refers to the role of gifted child.

'difficult'. I was concerned to see whether, as this was a largely primary school population, the children were taught by women teachers. The sex of the interviewer is known to affect the results of a test and it was important to relate the sex of the teachers to that of the pupil. If predominantly male pupils were being taught by predominantly female teachers, then it was possible that, as other studies have shown, women may have acted the 'schoolmistress' role and seen the boys as more difficult to manage that the girls on that account.

This was not found to be the case. In Britain nowadays, primary school teaching is becoming more and more a mixed sex profession. In addition, as there were a high number of private schools in the sample (30%) and these schools are very often single sex schools, the combination of factors was effective in such a way that each child was likely to be taught by a teacher of the same sex. It was the child's own classroom teacher who gave the opinion, so that boys' behaviours were not likely to be overly condemned by ladylike teachers. It was concluded that boys were indeed more difficult to have in the classroom and to live with at home.

Research reports very often fail to mention the sex of the investigatee and most often use males (or even rats) as subjects. These attempts to avoid the problems of sex differences result in either the subjects being treated as one undifferentiated mass, or the drawing of conclusions from data on males alone, which by assumption are then attributed to females also.

Achievement, for example, is an extremely important aspect of research with regard to gifted children, yet little investigation has been made into achievement motivation in females. In a review of research on achievement, Stein and Bailey (1973) concluded:

'First, like much psychological theory, achievement motivation theory was developed to explain the behaviour of males. Then attempts were made to use the theory for females. Not surprisingly it does not work for females.'

The effect of either regarding males and females as one, or of generalizing results from the male to apply to females, is that psychological theories are developed which are more suitable for males than females. Female behaviour is then seen as deviant or odd, while male behaviour is seen as normal.

Differences in the socialization of boys and girls in any culture are normally tied to the work that they are expected to do as adults. This is reflected in the role-duties which they are given as children. In Western culture, the nurturant mother role is actually a more full-time occupation for women than it is in any other culture. Temperamental differences between the sexes, in particular aggression and dependency, are doubly influenced in this way by tradition and future occupation. Aggression is associated with achievement, especially in Western culture, and is generally encouraged in boys and discouraged in girls (Barry *et al.*, 1957). Socialization differences affecting this one trait afford considerable explanation of the different behaviour of normal boys and girls in the classroom.

Where the parents believe them to be gifted, children are likely to be the subjects of intensified parental expectations. In my sample, twice as many boys as girls were considered to be gifted by their parents and although parental pressure on the children to achieve was higher than usual, it was equally high for both sexes. Parents of boys, however, said they expected them to stay longer in the educational system than parents of girls, though in fact the provision that girls received, e.g. of study space, was relatively better than for boys. The implications of parental expectations for boys would presumably make themselves felt as the children grow up to the age where they would go on into higher education. This may be judged by the proportions of boys and girls who apply for university-type education, i.e. fewer of the able girls.

## Achievement orientation

The most extensive work on the achievement motivation of boys has been carried out by McClelland and associates (McClelland *et al.*, 1953). They consider that achievement motivation is determined by the process of socialization, which is seen as an interaction between environment and heredity. The child, being socialized in this way, is considered to develop expectations about what any particular behaviour, such as talking or reading, will accomplish for him. He also takes pleasure (or positive reinforcement) from the demonstrated competence of these expectations, as long as they have a degree of uncertainty and the relevant cues are present. In this trial and error way, the child forms a frame of reference and discovers his own capabilities. If he does better than he anticipated, he will go on to attempt harder tasks, but if not, his standard will drop. However, parents' or teachers' encouragement must not be too high or too low, but just above the level of which the child is capable – the judgement is a fine one. The child is constantly building his own frame of reference from these experiences, but when the adult's (external) frame of reference is too strong, the child may fail to develop his own (internal) frame of reference adequately, which results in a dependency on adult estimation of his capability. Thus if the adult expectations are too high or are too difficult to sustain, the child must be a failure both in their eyes and in his own. Gifted children are always in danger of this kind of 'failure', which may be termed under-achievement.

McClelland gathered his original information by giving a projective test (TAT) to schoolboys in Japan, Germany, Brazil and India and to business executives or managers in Italy, Turkey and Poland. He then compared their results with those of American subjects. The TAT test is a series of less than clear pictures, into which the subject 'reads' a story. Assessment is then made of the content of the subject's story and it is that interpretation which provides the first great hazard. After that, there are translation errors, cultural influences, local school atmospheres, etc. which make the comparisons themselves a matter of subjective interpretation and therefore of doubtful validity. Nevertheless, this project has immensely stimulated the understanding of achievement orientation and has initiated much further research, supporting on the whole the original conclusions.

McClelland believes that children can and should be taught achievement motivation and that it is closely related to independence. Both achievement motivation and originality of thought are considered to derive from parent–child relationships that emphasise training for social independence. But there are pitfalls in the prescription:

(i)     Social independence does not always lead to high achievement motivation.

(ii)    Independence from parents does not always mean independence from others.

(iii)   Dependence may become the prime goal of achievement, as when the different children of a family compete for their parents' attention.

(iv)    Achievement motivation may result from a desire for dependence on others' opinions and is then of an immature form.

In fact, there are some forms of parental behaviour which are considered to act directly against achievement motivation:

(i)     Dominance by the father (not the mother) leads to a low level of self-reliance and low need for achievement in a son, who can't then work out high standards for himself.

(ii)    Low standards of excellence within the family and too much indulgence of the child.

(iii)   Too much protection encourages dependence. Early achievement motivation seems to demand that a son is thrown out of the nest before he is apparently ready to fly.

What is needed from parents are (McClelland, 1961):

'reasonably high standards of excellence imposed at a time when the sons can attain them, a willingness to attain them without interference, and real emotional pleasure in his achievements short of over-protection and indulgence'.

Freud anticipated this point of view, beautifully as always, in *A Childhood Recollection* (Freud *et al.* 1978):

'. . . if a man has been his mother's undisputed darling he retains throughout life the triumphant feelings, the confidence in success, which not seldom brings actual success along with it'.

In a study of the outcomes of general education in Ireland, Raven (1977) found that pupils of high achievement orientation held many attitudes and values which are usually considered to be middle-class. No matter what their social background actually was, their general attitudes were related to personal aspirations. Pupils bound for high status jobs were much more concerned to develop the abilities to work with others, to take initiative, to work for the good of their communities and to take responsibilities than were other pupils. Those bound for low status positions, whatever their origins, were much more concerned than others to be given strict rules to their lives and were much less keen to develop independence and initiative. The highly aspirant pupils were also the most keen to study hard at school, cut out the 'frills' of education and pass their examinations.

The psychological foundations of the upwardly-striving pupil appear at first glance to be sound. But Raven agrees with Berg (1970) in his research conclusions that extremely determined, highly achievement-orientated individuals are in fact destructive to organizations, in their thirst for personal gain. I suspect a dichotomy here between the world of education and the world of commerce. Outside a salaried employment it is difficult to run an organization destructively; the logical consequence would be that it would collapse. Clearly, big corporations run by hierarchies of power-hungry people rarely do collapse. But schools and hospitals, for example, are so supported by the community that individuals can indeed destroy their smooth running with relative impunity.

Probably because it is very difficult to measure, the innate components of achievement motivation have received very little attention.
However, there are other educationalists, notably **Piaget** (1971) who
interpret what may loosely be termed achievement motivation as an
inborn desire to right the balance of nature. For example, when a child is
given a new idea, she will seek to stabilize it in terms of the ideas which
she already has. This stabilizing activity is learning, which results in
achievement and the satisfaction from that activity then leads to a wish
for more of the same, constituting a type of achievement motivation. The
form that this new learning takes is obviously influenced by previous
experience.

## Sex differences in achievement orientation

McClelland's work is an attempt to separate the effects of achievement
motivation from those of intelligence. In a modified behaviourist sense,
his emphasis is on methods which emphasise early training for independence. This type of upbringing is usually given to boys and
sometimes to first-born and only girls. As far as American boys were
concerned, the team found three differences:

(i)     Male occupational choices can be treated as instances of 'risk
        taking'. Men typically do not choose fields in which their success
        is assured, but where it is possible. This 'risk taking' aspect of
        achievement motivation is probably an early divisor of boys' and
        girls' aspirations.

(ii)    Boys who score more highly on projective measures of achieve-
        ment motivation do better in school than boys with lower scores,
        but of the same ability.

(iii)   When boys believe their projective test material refers to their
        intelligence or leadership abilities, their concern with achieve-
        ment goes up.

But the evidence does not apply to girls, who are much more varied in
their endeavours to achieve. American girls, when asked about the
income they hoped to receive in payment for their expertise, have been
found to be relatively unambitious in comparison to their brothers.
They allotted far more importance to the nature of the work itself. Those
girls who wanted money did not expect to earn it themselves, but hoped
to acquire it through marriage (Turner, 1964).

Achievement orientation for young girls is not often the same as it is for boys, since they are normally expected to choose between a career and their own family; it is unusual for women to be eminently successful at both. A good deal of energy and time is taken up in most girls' secondary school years with preparing for, if not securing, a husband, and the competition for involvement in a girl's life by school is often lost. Boys marry at a relatively older age than girls and acquire more education and career training before the event. But it is during adolescence that future career choices, in the broad sense of what to concentrate on and what to leave out, are being made.

In American high schools (of mixed sex), Coleman (1961) found that girls of higher intelligence avoided being outstanding scholars and in every school the girl who was thought to be the 'best scholar' by her peers was less bright than the boys who were so known. In other words, the brighter girls who were capable of doing the best work had managed to conceal their intellectual assets from those around them, while those pupils who were regarded as scholars were less than the best (Kipnis, 1976). Headmistresses of girls' schools in Britain have long claimed that the best chance of academic success that a girl has is in a girls-only school. As a child in Canada, I well remember the shame at having done better than the boys in my class. Girls in competition with boys do not always find it satisfactory to be the winners.

Since 1972, Professor Julian Stanley has been running a mathematical holiday camp for 'mathematically precocious youth' as a spin-off from his research at Johns Hopkins University, Baltimore (Stanley, Keating and Fox, 1974). A colleague of Stanley's, Dr Lynn Fox has analyzed the reluctance of girls to recognize their mathematical gifts. She believes that girls are still being steered away from such a masculine subject in the schools and that consequently they are often ashamed to admit that they are good at maths; it only invites ridicule and dislike. She quotes one girl denying that she was going to a camp for gifted children, but claimed that it was for *remedial* maths instead. Fox observed that girls more often say that maths is a useless subject practically and that it won't help them get jobs. Naturally, there is a high drop-out rate for girls in this subject and they seem to derive less benefit from the course.

Many studies, such as those of Stott (1945) and Douglas (1968) found that while parents encouraged sons to take jobs for which they were not suited in various ways, daughters were pressurized to take jobs which were generally below their ability. In my study of gifted children, the boys were expected to stay on at school longer than girls. Education was also considered to be more important for a boy's future than for that of a girl. As my evidence was taken from educationally highly motivated parents, there are probably more extreme differences in parents' attitudes towards the education of their sons and daughters in the general population.

## Socialization in the family

The family is crucial in the social development of children. Although there are many changing forms of family life, the prime responsibility for rearing children in almost every society is still, by law and custom, the prerogative of the family. The biggest recent change in family life has probably been in the differing roles of mothers and fathers. However, as the family does continue to provide the most effective socializing function that a child is ever likely to encounter, it is seen here in terms of its present, if transient, culture.

The family group into which a child is born begins the socialization process. It is concerned, for example, with teaching the ways in which one's sex, or the people in one's geographical area, behave, as well as the place of such behaviour in the greater society outside. School and community continue the process together, since education is not just an instruction but an influential part of emotional and behavioural development. Socialization must take place through communication, which is the most important force in family life. If messages are unclear or contradictory, communication will be inadequate and can produce confusion and conflict. Good communication undoubtedly smooths the socialization process for the children of any family, but messages can, in a sense, be too clear. When a child is directed without choice into a way of behaving which is not acceptable, then he is likely to show signs of frustration, such as behaviour which is difficult for others to live with.

It is often considered that gifted children, placed in the position where they are expected to behave and think like normal children, are victims of such a situation. Either at home or in school, if a gifted child is fettered by convention and rigid upbringing - in a mould which does not fit - he may just break out. Because of the rigid situation which brought this about in the first place, any nonconforming signs which the child shares may be considered unacceptable by the parents (see Chapter 4).

Communication in a family must be a two-way process. It is not only the children, but the parents also who have to be aware and to learn from each other. It is often asked whether the parents (or teacher) of a gifted child need to be gifted themselves in order to communicate. In fact, parents of gifted children, except in rare cases, have an ability level which is similar to the child's. Where there is a blood tie, common characteristics are normally present to a significant extent between those who share it. Teachers, of course, do not share such a tie, but by virtue of their qualifications, they are well into the higher ability ranges themselves. This question will be referred to again in more detail in Chapter 5.

## Two-way socialization

It is simply not possible to ask a baby what his hopes and intentions are. Maybe under hypnosis or in deep psychological analysis an adult can remember being a baby, but such remembrances are difficult to distinguish from imagination and from what we have been told by others. It is safer to assume that we cannot see into a baby's mind or know how it feels to be a baby, but we can observe how a baby acts and causes reactions within the family. It is only by backward deduction from a baby's behaviour, particularly with one close adult – his mother – that clues can be obtained as to what is going on. But whatever aspects of a baby's behaviour may be deduced as intentional must be in accordance with his known biological development and level of functioning. Indeed, recent work indicates that the 'special' relationship a baby has with his mother, on which the child's functioning as a socially competent human being eventually depends, is itself founded on the known stages of biological development.

Right from the beginning, the infant has an active part to play and his mother allots him a role as a person. This person has needs, wishes and intentions, which are often verbalized for him by his mother – 'Ah, you want a nice drink then', 'Is that chair comfortable for you?' etc. But the process of mental growth is not something imposed on a passive infant. If his system was merely reactive, it would not grow, change and acquire concepts, intentions, or the capacities for communication, as in fact it does.

A baby is not a piece of machinery but an organism that develops through interactions with others. He is born 'striving' and 'experimenting' (Gauld and Shotter, 1977) not consciously perhaps, but functioning nevertheless. He has a very complex world to sort out and usually has the means available with which to strive and experiment; he interacts with the world in the form of his mother and he is stimulated by and can use toys. Using such devices, he can try out different strategies, and see which are worth repeating. It is not only the psychologist who implies that the baby is striving and experimenting; primarily it is the mother who does it all the time. Because she sees her baby as a growing person, he comes to behave in time in ways which are consistent with this and comes to have intentions, concepts, etc.

Mothers introduce their babies into their own culture, such as one would do for a helpless foreigner. In her attempts to bring him into the cultural picture, she establishes a 'dialogue' with him and to do this, she is sensitive to what her baby initiates, as well as suggesting and demanding certain behaviours from him. She encourages the activities of which she approves, discourages those she considers inappropriate, tries to extend the baby's grasp of what is appropriate, and is sensitive to signs, which she can reinforce, that he is understanding what is wanted of him. It is not just behaviour that she is working on, but a total conceptual and physical learning system. The baby–mother dialogue is most certainly a two-way process, its success depending on the sensitivity and tolerance of both parties; neither can remain unaffected. The normal child becomes a smaller version of the adults in his family, while the mother, by putting into action her *assumption* that the child is creatively intelligent, becomes a skilled applied psychologist.

Recent studies have shown that mothers treat their babies like human beings from the moment of birth. Macfarlane (1974) has observed how mothers are quick to see the personal aspects of their new baby. For his part, the baby's capacity for eye-to-eye contact with the mother has been found to be a key factor in the development of attachment to him. The forerunner of this capacity is the infant's state of visual alertness; newborn babies differ in how often they spontaneously become alert and how quickly they respond with alertness to the mother's care. Gesell (1950) states that gifted children show this capacity from birth and many parents of gifted children say the same thing.

## Very early sensitivity

From very early on, babies begin to imitate speech movement patterns with their lips and also imitate large body movements. Within seconds of birth, babies can detect the direction of a sound and turn to face it. Twelve hours after birth, babies can detect the difference between human speech and other sounds, reacting with imperceptible rhythmic movements, which show up on slow-motion film. Fourteen-day-old babies are capable of imitating expressions and finger movements of an adult sitting by them. Videotape is often used in these observations, since repetition of a sequence gives much greater clarity. Using this technique, the Newsons (1976) found considerable reflection of body and face movements between young babies and their mothers. In their words:

> '... different sensori-motor components of the infants' activity are highly synchronized with each other ... his action sequences are temporally organized so that they can mesh – with a high degree of precision – with similar patterns of action produced by the human caretakers.'

Thus, mother and baby can be seen to work in harmony. It is not a perfect, but a changing relationship, each communicator alternating with and in a sense teaching the other in rhythmic sequence (Schaffer, 1974). Mother and baby can 'talk' and 'listen' to one another, but if mother is short on either the talking or the listening, the baby fails to develop as well as it might do otherwise.

In America, Brazelton (1975) has used a split-screen technique to record on videotape simultaneously an interacting mother and infant during the first four months of life. The tape shows a remarkable choreography of two human beings responding instinctively and sensitively to each other. Unless the mother is sensitive to this cyclical pattern, Brazelton says, she may overload her baby's capacity for prolonged attention. The baby's response to such overloading is to show only brief periods of attention and prolonged periods of non-attention.

As they grow, infants becoming children come to know that adults appreciate signs that the children understand what they are doing in the same terms as the adult. A smile, a moment of shared gaze, or an affectionate remark may serve this purpose. Styles of mothering can be seen to have a definite effect on the child's mental development, while in the course of growth, children continue to shape their parents. For example, American studies over many years have found a relationship between restrictiveness on the part of the parents and dependency in the child. However the findings of Bell and Ainsworth (1972) reversed the conclusion of earlier workers that the child who was restricted fails to develop skills to act independently. In fact, the relationship is the reverse; if the child is independent by nature, then the parents follow by being less restrictive. Babies' individual sleep patterns also affect their relationship with parents; they evoke contrasting reactions of calm and frustration – emotions which in turn are passed on to the infant. These sleep patterns arise through a variety of influences, such as the circumstances of pregnancy, birth and early parental care.

A reflex type of physiological arousal may come before a proper relationship develops between a newborn baby and an adult. It is often noted in nurseries, for example, that babies will cry in response to the sound of other babies crying, but whether they take up each others' cries out of empathy or by an arousal of the nervous system is unknown.

It is doubtful whether high intellectual ability benefits social relationships in either children or adults. Some investigators have reported age-related changes in positive social behaviour, i.e. the older the child (in early childhood), the more social her behaviour. A recent study by Abroms *et al.* (1979) found that parents who were easy-going tended to have children showing more mature social skills; they reported that among gifted three-year-olds, a high IQ proved to be the best predictive measure of positive social behaviour. But a period of time in nursery school tended to iron out the advantage of IQ as a predictor of social skills.

Much of the understanding of this very early parent–child interaction has been discovered within the last few years and is not always recognized by older texts on child development. It is surely here, at the very beginning of life, that those babies who are to become gifted children take their first gulps of learning. Lack of early stimulation is difficult, though not impossible to make up for later, since the repressed, unstimulated child begins by failing to bring about teaching responses in adults. The babies of sensitive, educated, happy parents on the other hand obviously have a great deal going for them.

## Birth order and family size

Over the years, a considerable amount of evidence has accumulated showing that the position in which a child is born into a family affects both her intellect and personality. Most notably, it affects her level of achievement, but almost all the research on effects of birth order has been American. In a review of all the work to date, Sutton-Smith and Rosenberg (1970) drew particular attention to the many studies which found differences in the attitudes of parents towards first-born, as compared with other children.

First-born children have all their parents' attention for a while and of course each is the one on which a new set of parents try out their child-raising skills. Because they are first-born, parents may well have unrealistic expectations of what those babies should be able to do. It has been found that mothers of first-borns expected far more than they did of later-born children and they also encouraged and helped them more. This behaviour in the mother slowly but surely affects the child's level of achievement and character. Fathers probably behave like that too, but their interactions with their first-borns have gone largely unmeasured.

A study of 400 000 young men conscripted into the Dutch Army (Belmont and Marolla, 1973) found that the birth order of the men was significantly related to their intelligence test scores. The higher the birth order, the higher the score. This research found that first-born men had the highest scores, second-born the next highest and so on, but only children scored less highly than first-borns. This birth order effect appeared at all social and economic levels, throughout the great numbers of young men involved.

It appeared therefore that intelligence dropped with later birth order and consequently the larger the family, the lower the intelligence of the younger children. One might conclude from this, as Insel and Lindgren (1978) did, that large families have a depressing effect on mental development. They suggest that the more children there are in a family, the greater the strain on the intellectual resources available and the less each subsequent child receives. This effect is essentially due to the 'crowding' in the family situation.

Several surveys have found a similar correlation between family size and poor achievement. Nisbet and Entwistle (1967) and Douglas (1968) came to the same conclusions about English families and interpreted their results as being due to socio-economic rather than inherited influences. In other words, the poor tended to have more children than the rich and were accordingly short of those environmental influences which promote intellectual growth. But it is possible that influences greater than the immediate family circumstances are at work.

In an investigation into educational attainment in Eire, Cullen (1969) made a different discovery. There was no marked difference between the sizes of families of educationally advanced and educationally retarded children. Most importantly, though, this situation only held before the arrival of the sixth child. Eire is a Catholic country, where birth control is largely forbidden. Cullen suggests that six children could represent the point at which decisions to limit family size, without transgressing religious principles, would be noticeable. She found that it was not the size of the family, but the attitudes and expectations of the parents concerning education which were important in school achievement.

All other studies of the effects of birth order have been carried out on children born into culturally heterogeneous societies, such as North

America. But family size is not necessarily a matter of chance. In countries where there is a big gulf in the standard of living between rich and poor, a large family may be a display of wealth on the one hand, or alternatively a source of free labour. In those circumstances, families at either end of the economic spectrum would have larger families than those in the middle. This effect could be seen in nineteenth-century Britain and North America and is found in South America today. It would not be expected that the large families of the rich would suffer from intellectual deprivation, but, as yet, the abilities of rich children have not been studied.

First and second-borns were studied, with their mothers, by Lasko (1954) in their own homes, between the ages of one and nine years. The first-born children did in fact receive much more attention in their first two years than the second-borns. Although first-borns were treated less warmly by their parents than the second-borns, by the age of three or four they were still expected to achieve more highly. Other studies have also found that parents continue to expect more of their first-born child than later-born ones for many years. This remains true even though the parents may realize that their earlier expectations had been unrealistic.

First-born children seem to model themselves more on their parents than later-borns and are thereby more conservative by nature than their siblings. They also seem to be more sensitive and aware of other peoples' feelings, which may be due to their having adopted adult values at an early age. Only children, who are first-born and last-born, are not quite the same as the first-born child of a family; they are even more dependent and highly achieving and also have a higher level of self-confidence. In comparison to first-born children, they are more aggressive and less anxious, but also more obedient to their parents.

Middle children have proverbially always had a hard time, squashed between the others. Sutton-Smith and Rosenberg suggest that this is actually true and that they do receive less attention than the other children. As a consequence, they are more likely to use unattractive means of gaining attention, such as quarrelling or being obstinate. They are often the least popular members of the family.

As far as popularity with friends is concerned, last-borns come top of the list, followed by middles, while the least popular are the first-borns. Teachers tend to agree with this hierarchy and show the same relative amounts of friendliness to the different birth order children, from kindergarten right through to school leaving, as other children do.

Children who are born into different positions in a family are not, in reality, born into the same family make-up. Add a change of sex to the possible differences resulting from birth order and the new baby's life may be very different indeed to the last one's. But there must always be a first-born child in a family and with the average size of the Western family getting smaller, there are relatively more first-borns than there were. In some countries, where one-child families are common, there should be a preponderance of only-child characteristics among children, but this possibility has not been tested scientifically.

The children in my study who were designated gifted by their parents contained 13% only children and 56% first-born; together, these form 69%, i.e. over two-thirds of the sample. The control group, which contained children who were of similar ability, but not designated gifted by their parents, had only 52% first-born and only children. The random control group had only 37% first-born and only children.

The first group of children were undoubtedly high achievers, were described by their parents as difficult to bring up and were not very popular with friends or teachers at school. The third group had very few of these characteristics and contained less than half the first group's number of first-born and only children. The conclusion that the behaviour and achievement of the first group had something to do with their birth order is tempting. Terman (1925) found a similarly high proportion of first-born and only children in his sample of gifted children and their studies have reported the same. It can at least be said that being born a first or only child will increase a baby's chances of being gifted and 'difficult'.

## Friendship

The urge to be sociable, to relate to others, is apparent from the earliest stages of a child's existence. From birth, the mother obviously fills the most important social need of her baby, but as he grows, so does his appetite for contact with others. Humans have a basic hunger for companionship, for emotional support and for a sense of belonging to society. Differentiation as a person from mother begins at about the age of two, but for another year or two afterwards, the infant plays alongside, rather than with other children. From then, friends come onto the scene and it is these early relationships with friends that can be seen later, reflected in the way he adjusts to other people.

Many of the lists of characteristics describing gifted children state (as do many of their parents) that such children have difficulty in making friends, especially of their own age-group. The way that a child gets on with his friends may be a very sensitive diagnostic indicator of development. When a child does not become involved with his age-group and is not comfortable in their activities, there is reason to believe that something is wrong. This does assume, though, that there are peers about that he *could* relate to.

American research by Hartup and Lougee (1975) and by Roff and Sells (1968) found that poor relationships with peers often presaged mental health problems in later life. Roff found that he could predict adult behaviour with great accuracy from a subject's childhood friendships. He concluded this from years of follow-up studies, using a control group, both groups having come to his notice during his work at a child guidance clinic. All the children had been sent to him for behaviour problems occuring both at home and at school, but it was only those who were considered as likeable by their peers who overcame these difficulties in adult life.

Social adjustment begins very early in life and it is possible to judge from the outset whether it is going smoothly or not. Another follow-up study by Cowen and associates (1973) at Rochester University found that other children were very adept at spotting maladjustment in all its forms. They proved to be very sensitive in this and were able to identify children who were later to become disturbed in adolescence and adulthood.

A child's future well-being is very often tied to his peer relationships (Hartup, 1975):

> 'There are some necessities in children's development that require interaction with coequals – that is individuals who have the same kind of development status and competencies in the cognitive and social areas as they do.'

Accumulating evidence of the vital importance of peers to a child for his future stability is particularly significant for the highly able child. It is only through a child's relationship with friends whom he can respect that it is possible for him to learn the shape of future behaviour. This will include sexual expression, aggressive conduct, ethical behaviour and even the overcoming of disabling fears and anxieties and gaining a sense of emotional security. Thus, a child's friends are more than just playmates; they are essential to his development. It is when he has no friends that problems are likely to arise in social development and since many of the children in my target group were said to have few friends (83%) as compared with the control groups (30%), it is very possible that some of the behaviour disturbances they showed were for that reason. It is hard to know which comes first – that children do not make friends because their peers find them unattractive, or (as it is often said) that gifted children refuse to make friends because they find it too difficult to communicate with their peers. The reasons usually given for this situation are firstly that their intellects are so superior they find other children boring and secondly that their language development is so advanced they find it frustrating to talk to others of the same age. As a consequence, they keep to themselves and find themselves solitary things to do, resulting in the gifted child's reputation for isolation.

There is very little British evidence about the influence of age-group peers on a child; researchers have mentioned it almost in passing and mostly in a negative sense. Thus, in studies of delinquent children, peers can be seen to be a 'bad influence' on a good child, but even these anecdotal accounts indicate that the positive effect of a child's friends works to enhance self-esteem and confirm moral standards. The parents in Clark's study of Young Fluent Readers (Clark, 1976) saw nursery education as having more than an educational function. It was valued as a place where these bright children could go to play with others of their own age, when there were none available at home. But of those parents who did keep their children at home:

> 'Several parents remarked that had their child been less willing to concentrate and more troublesome, or yearned for further company, then they might have thought differently'.

The likelihood is, then, that the more 'difficult' children were the ones who were sent to nursery schools although few of these children were described by their parents as not being liked by other children. Both the parents and the teachers agreed that unpopular children tended to be rather solitary, but the adults considered it to be the result of self-sufficiency on the part of those children, rather than their being shunned by others.

Bettleheim (1969) has described children brought up on certain types of kibbutz (collective settlement) in Israel, where they live with peers, rather than their parents. The infant leaves its parents on the fourth day of life and lives in the Children's House with a small number of the same age-group. Multiple mothering takes place since the child's own parents spend some time each day with it, but quality of relationship is considered to be more important than quantity. The infant does not have the security of the one-to-one relationship, but neither will it have the extremes of non-mutality, taking its 'emotional input' by way of the professional nurse, peers and parents. Although a 'flatness' of the kibbutz personality has been remarked upon, these children learn early to interact with many others, which may contribute to personal independence. But other reports say they are over-dependent on the approval of their peers; high social value is placed on the group and on collective emotional experience. Individualism is not encouraged and perhaps because of this, few gifted artists, writers or musicians have so far been produced from the kibbutz milieu.

Children learn to cope with their feelings of aggression in the course of interactions with friends, rather than with families. Much of the evidence for this comes from animal research. In his very extensive and lengthy studies of primates, Harlow (1969) showed that it is through peer relationships that young animals build up a repertoire of effective and acceptable aggressive behaviours, as well as other ways of dealing with aggressive feelings. Jane van Lawick-Goodall (1971), having spent many years observing the natural behaviour of chimpanzees in Africa, described very graphically the value of the rough and tumble of the young in learning how far to go.

The stumbling block in learning how to cope with aggression within the family is that a child's relationship with his parents is complex, but still basically one of a subordinate to an authority; child to parent, in fact. Children who are constantly hostile or unusually timid in school, for instance, may well have lacked exposure to interactions which teach youngsters how to express, as well as control, aggressive urges. From his years of research on the nature of peer interactions, Hartup found that peer modelling is among the most powerful of the social influences to which children are ever exposed. These influences begin in the toddler years, are intensified at nursery school and continue through life. Peer modelling can enable a child to function either within or outside the rules of society, but, as always, the impact of the environment is tempered by the child's own nature.

From the outset of his lifetime's work, Piaget (1968) found that much of a child's moral understanding developed from the kind of interactions he had with his peers. Young children are prisoners of their own perspective, 'egocentric' in Piaget's term. Only later, when they begin to interact with peers, do children learn how to behave in the larger society outside the home. It is his peers who will enable a child to gain a sense of social perspective - to see life from another's point of view and to be concerned with others. Criticism and support are often acceptable from a friend when they are not from a parent and when with their friends, children know they are not wrestling alone with family problems.

47

Feelings of isolation, sexual inadequacy and aggression are the common lot of children, and can be shared between friends.

Several American researchers, notably Bandura (1967) and Hartup and Lougee (1975) believe that peer influence works largely by the modelling process. Bandura demonstrated this with a group of children who were afraid of dogs. One of them, who was not afraid, was asked to play with a dog while the others watched. Those children who had seen the 'model' playing with the dog were then significantly less fearful of dogs than the control group, who had not witnessed this modelling process. But children who do not play with other children may become sad and inward looking. They may find it increasingly difficult to make normal contact with others, a problem which only exacerbates the downward spiral, until they learn to become social isolates and appear not to 'need' others of their own age. Also for many parents, other children that their child may mix with are a threat. They do not want their child to imitate behaviour of which they would disapprove, or experience the force of a peer group, possibly to be directed against their own wishes. Thus parents and peers form two very complex and contrasting forces acting on the life of a child.

It is the quality of a child's emotional ties with his family which determines how much influence his friends will have over him. Insecure children are more likely than secure children to turn for support outside the family. The extent of peer group influence is also affected by the culture; in some cultures, family is 'all' and outsiders have very little influence, even after they marry into it. Hartup sees the two forces – parents and peers – as complementary, rather than antagonistic; sometimes the family is essential to good development and sometimes the peer group. He argues that peer modelling effects are usually good and that parents' fears of the bad influence of their children's friends are not usually justified. It is perhaps the over-conscientious parent who supposes that only his influences will be the suitable ones and that the child would be better off without the others which life may hold. Parents are, as always, the models for adulthood and this is not a small consideration when peer groups seem to threaten. However parents can also be sensitive to and involved with their children's friends, who are essential for childhood socialization and personal development.

## Discordant families

All families have a measure of discord somewhere. On the whole people learn to live with it, but sometimes the tension and problems become so intolerable that the result is divorce or separation. Though it is difficult to disentangle the effects of rumbling disharmony and a parental split, there is an undoubted relationship between discordant family relationships and problem behaviour in the children, especially boys. This is the result both of the strain within the family and also of possible resultant animosity of parents towards the child. It is the disturbance in the family which causes children to be unhappy, not the other way round; children do not often make their families discordant because of their inherent problem behaviour. As family life becomes more harmonious, the behaviour of the children improves (Rutter, Quinton and Yule, 1976). However, children who are severely handicapped, either mentally or physically, can bring about considerable stress in the family. It is also conceivable, although there is no firm evidence on this point, that a gifted child in a non-gifted family may have a continuously disturbing effect.

Tension between parents affects the way in which they bring up their children; the quality of general supervision will suffer. Punishment given in a warm, stable relationship is effective if it is close in time to the offence and it is not then normally detrimental to the recipient. But in a state of tension, punishment may become erratic, whether it is the favoured middle-class punishment of the withdrawal of love, or the more common, sharp physical communication. It is the inconsistency of ineffective control which is significant emotionally and which may result in the development of aggressive behaviour.

The reverse situation in which parents are overly anxious and protective of their children can be equally damaging to a child's normal development. The anxious solicitude which accompanies such over-control communicates itself to a child and results in his becoming anxious about himself. This childhood anxiety can become quite a habit so that the child learns to behave in an anxious, or even 'neurotic' manner, even though the anxiety producers – his parents – may be absent.

An example of this over-anxious behaviour was discovered by myself when collecting my first sample of children whose parents had joined the association for gifted children. Virtually all the parents of children aged over 14 refused to allow them to take part in the study; indeed, I was warned not to approach the children directly in spite of my protestations that I would not consider such an action. The reason invariably given was that the child was entering on an examination course and must not be distracted. Although I explained that my intervention would take up no more than two hours, many parents agreed to be interviewed themselves only as long as their child remained unaware of the research. In England, a national examination – the General Certificate of Education at Ordinary level – is taken usually between 15 and 17 years of age. Success in this allows pupils to proceed to the Advanced level, hence its importance. In contrast parents of younger children, who were not examination-bound, were very helpful. Fear of a two-hour intervention out of school hours in a two-year course can only be considered as over-anxiety.

Depression is particularly frequent among mothers of young children in urban areas (Brown and Harris, 1978); reasons most often given are loneliness, change of role and lack of self-esteem. The mother's capacity to respond to the child's emotional and intellectual needs becomes adversely affected and then the child of an unhappy, withdrawn mother is in a stressful, frustrating situation which may itself induce aggressive or withdrawn behaviour. There is also evidence that emotional disorders in children happen more frequently in only children or children of small families (Rutter, Tizard and Whitmore, 1970), but that some employment outside the home goes a long way towards relieving the mother's depression. Mothers of the most stable children in my sample were most likely to work outside the home.

Parents may be trying to produce a child whose excellence showers credit on them and if the baby fails to live up to their expectations, he is seen as letting them down. But if the child's own needs are ignored, he will fail to gain confidence in his own abilities and perhaps try to become the person he imagines is wanted. Fromm (1941), giving the psycho-analytical view, refers to this as 'dynamic adaption' and gives the example of a boy who submits to the commands of his strict and threatening father, being too much afraid of him to do otherwise, and becomes a 'good' boy. He adapts to the necessities of the situation, but something happens to him; he may develop an intense hostility against his father, which he represses, since it would be too dangerous to express it, or even be aware of it.

> 'This repressed hostility . . . is a dynamic factor in his character structure. It may create new anxiety and thus lead to still deeper submission; it may set up a vague defiance, directed against no one in particular but rather toward life in general . . .'

Parents who behave in this over-demanding way tend to suffer from a severe lack of self-esteem. Due to their own background, they expect to be let down; therefore they are afraid of making friends and may appear distant, elusive and hostile. As a result, they tend to be lonely and socially very isolated. Their expectations of their children are tied up with their own life experiences, which are most likely to have been perceived by themselves as unhappy. Some parents may feel they had had a raw deal in their own upbringing; in my sample, 14% of the mothers who had joined the National Association for Gifted Children were dissatisfied or bitter about their own education, whereas on average 2% of the mothers of the control groups felt this.

The reverse situation arises when these parents' own parents were perceived as having had unrealistic expectations of them and now, as parents themselves, they are repeating their own upbringing by making the same demands on their own children. The centre of the problem is that the expectations they make cannot be fulfilled because they are unrealistic (Renvoize, 1975). Parents who believe their children to be gifted are most likely to fall into this trap of having expectations which are too high. Even if a child is truly gifted in any sense, he will find it difficult to be gifted in every respect all the time. A child who is not gifted, but believed to be so, must necessarily disappoint his parents most of the time, with consequent emotional problems. Those children in my sample who were described by their parents as gifted – whether they were or not – had a very much higher level of behaviour disturbance, as described by their parents and teachers, than other equally able children.

The causes of marital disharmony are many and varied, but it is often helpful for the disturbed children of such marriages if the reasons for the growth of tension can be discovered. For example, marriages between very young people tend to break down relatively quickly; a new relationship and the process of parenting involve considerable stress and those affected by it may need much support to survive these difficult years. In addition, the relative poverty and consequent accommodation problems which are often experienced then add to their tension and anger. Sometimes there is an irreversible clash of personalities, while problems of expectation, role-behaviour, attitudes and values are fairly common.

It is well recognized that social learning is more readily accomplished in a home which is low in tension. Children find it difficult to acquire normal social values and show appropriate behaviour when the atmosphere in which they live is emotionally charged. Also, where parents find it difficult to cope with one another, they will find themselves less able to attend to the emotional needs of their children. The situation can become circular and frustrating, and one common result of frustration is aggression. A child is particularly likely to become aggressive if either or both parents provide him with an adult model of aggressive behaviour. The child accomplishes his modelling by imitation and identification (Bandura, 1967), but fortunately a child may also model himself on the one parent with whom he has a good relationship (Rutter, 1972).

When the relationship between parents and child has been good, the death of a parent has a less disastrous effect on the child than a marital split; emotional disturbance and antisocial behaviour are less likely. It is important to distinguish between the children of one-parent families who are in that position because of the death of a parent and those who are in it for other reasons. Children can identify with a loved person who has died or from whom they have been separated; they may then incorporate real or imagined features of the person in an attempt to be close again.

The National Children's Bureau (Ferri, 1976) have found that behavioural and educational handicaps suffered by children in one-parent families are more likely to be associated with problems of poverty, housing and social class than with specific loss of a mother or father. The sample was national (UK) of 750 children at eleven years old, but unfortunately the age of the loss of the parent was not shown, nor whether certain children had in fact always had only one parent. This is important, as emotional strain and later personality disorders are more likely to have been experienced if the child was then under five, or if the lost parent was of the same sex as the child.

## Socialization in schools

Since schools first existed, it has been an important part of their function to socialize pupils; they often call it 'making responsible citizens'. Many parents, too, see the school as the first place in which their children will learn how to become members of the community. It is in the classroom and the playground that children come into contact for the first time with authority outside the home. The nature of the attitudes that the child learns there are part of the basis of his ultimate adaptation and adjustment to the world beyond the school gates.

Recently, there has been a growth of research on normal children actually carried out in the school situation, rather than in psychological laboratories or through purely theoretical considerations. Little research has been done on gifted children in the school situation, other than my own, at least in Britain, but the climate of opinion is changing and more investigation is planned. It has been found that many schools restrict social growth and over-emphasise conformity, i.e. they have a negative as well as a positive influence on children. Exceptional children – a category which includes gifted as well as disadvantaged children – may do least well at schools which enforce rigid social norms that are alien to them.

Many writers, among them John Holt (1969) and Ivan Illich (1970), have drawn attention to these problems and there has also been practical research, both in America and in Britain, which shows up the particular failings of certain rigid types of schools (Wiseman, 1964; Silberman, 1970). However, most research evidence refers to children's academic achievement rather than the interpersonal processes which mould children in schools, for example Bennett's work on formal and informal teaching (Bennett, 1976), which measured achievement by paper and pencil tests and ignored broader educational issues. But although classroom research has been growing considerably during the last decade, especially in America, very little real understanding has emerged of its effects on the mental health of children. In addition, there is a danger of isolating the classroom from society, which must be a false situation.

It is certainly difficult to quantify socialization processes in schools. Time sampling is a frequently used method in which the researcher sits at the back of a class with a stopwatch; every half minute or so, certain specific behaviours of teachers and members of the class are noted and ticked on a check list. In this way, a picture of a class's activity can be built up over time. Videotapes are even more valuable, as they can be played back many times and the actions depicted on them can be quantified, which gives much greater freedom of observation.

As yet, however, no researcher has shown that children's behaviour problems have emanated specifically from school, a conclusion which would imply that there is no complementary family behaviour also having a causal effect in individual cases. If the causes of troubled behaviour in children do start in the school, then it might be expected that members of the same school or class, as a group, would show evidence of that trouble. But in fact, children in any situation where they might be so affected show considerable variation of behaviour. Clearly, children respond very differently to individual teachers and school settings.

The impact that a child's daily school experience has on his evolving interpersonal strengths and weakness has been too much neglected by researchers. It is especially in school that children's perceptions of their capacities and competence take hold; they learn to recognize their self-image and begin to behave according to it. The single and longest lasting effect that a school has on its pupils is in how it affects their self-concepts. The whole system, but especially the teachers, has the potential to make or mar the way pupils will think about themselves for life. Children do not enter school as passive dolls, but as individuals, who have already had their share of emotional distress and traumas in the outside world.

In an experiment to test whether teachers' attitudes changed children's abilities, Rosenthal and Jacobson (1968) gave intelligence tests to a class of young pupils. They told the teachers the names of the brightest 20% in their class. These children had in fact been chosen at random, but the results appeared to affect the attitudes of the teachers so that they behaved differently towards their 'brightest' students. At the end of the year, this 20% of children did in fact come to be measured as being at the top of the class. The researchers concluded that the amazing change in the children's measured IQ could only have been brought about by the altered attitudes of the teachers. Unfortunately, no one has managed to reproduce this famous experiment and their original statistics are open to question. Among many others, Finn (1972) and Thorndike (1968) have criticised the study on methodological lines, while Beez (1968) and Claiborn (1969) tried to replicate it, but un-successfully. The book containing these results caused quite a stir in the educational world at the time and may have so disillusioned other teachers that the experiment could not be reproduced until the original one has been forgotten.

Using videotape to study the means by which a teacher interacts with his class, teachers' expectations are seen to affect whom they select to answer questions, whom they allow to stumble in search for an answer and whom they never involve. Chaikin and his associates (1974) found that teachers who expected a superior performance from their pupils used many more positive non-verbal behaviours, such as smiling, leaning towards the pupil, making eye contact and nodding the head, than they did with pupils of whom they expected less. Chaikin's conclusion was that the teacher did not need to put his image of the pupil into words; the message was there, in subtle yet potent ways. The information which is slowly accumulating about teachers' influence on pupils shows how considerable is this effect, which occurs for several hours each day in term-time. Multiply this many times, as happens when several teachers agree in the staff-room on their policy towards certain children, and the outcome must be very effective indeed.

The dual home/school effect on children's behaviour has been documented by only a few researchers, notably the Newsons in Britain (Newson and Newson, 1977) and Zax and Cowen (1969) in America. The Newsons' study was very thorough and included visiting the children's homes, which I did myself in an earlier piece of work (Freeman, 1974), as well as in that described in the present book. In the 1974 research, I was investigating (among other things) the effects of home and school on aesthetic achievement in children. I found that both home and school were able to initiate interest, but it was only where the home was entirely supportive that the child could be put in the category of 'aesthetically talented'. This type of in-depth research cannot be done when the researcher makes no attempt to visit the children's homes.

Some psychologists have taken children into clinics to judge their relationships with others; for instance Love and Kaswan (1974) in their large investigation of children with behaviour problems. They believed that examining children under clinical conditions was more 'direct, detailed and controlled' than it would have been in their homes, or in schools (where data were also collected). No doubt it was, but it would also be barren in other respects for lack of interaction in the real-life setting.

The effects of selecting children for different teaching groups and learning experiences are examined in Chapter 5.

## THE GREATER SOCIETY

Until the 1960s, there was little attempt made to look at the wide range of cultural environments which exist in the world from the point of view of learning. Certainly, few studies have tried to control genetic factors across the cultural groups so that the differences between what is learned and what is inborn might be distinguished. Social behaviour is most often assumed to be learned, but in fact we know very little about the relationship between the physical and social environments. In fact over the years psychologists seem to have made two great assumptions about the social behaviour of different people. Firstly that all people are much the same, that is like the Western world, and secondly that people who are not like the Western world are so odd as to be considered abnormal.

55

It is the West, in particular the USA, which has provided the 'norm' for the world. But even within the Western population such relatively minor differences in environment as class and sex can be seen to be effective in influencing individual behaviour. How much greater must the influence be from radically different cultures?

## Normality and deviance

The word 'abnormal' is often taken to mean something bad. To call someone abnormal is usually to involve an uncomplimentary tone; it may imply a degree of mental disturbance, a physical problem, or an insinuation of immorality. It makes assumptions of value in a negative sense.

On the other hand 'normal' can be used to describe what is believed to be right within a particular society; not being normal produces unhappiness, whereas if you are normal you fit into prevailing concepts of what is right and what is wrong. It is only recently, though, that the moral values which have been attached to such words have come under systematic scrutiny and the consequent freedom from moral judgement has enabled social science research to proceed in leaps and bounds. For instance, we do not (as scientists) regard the beating of children as being right or wrong, but we do identify the results of this action. Nor should we regard gifted children as a socially determined elite, though many people do. Moral judgement is always inherently present, but in the interests of objectivity, we try to exclude it from the results of scientific enquiry. Lemert, a sociologist, defined social problems merely as situations 'about which a large number of people feel disturbed and unhappy – this and nothing more' (Lemert, 1951). His main focus of interest lay in the processes whereby problems were socially recognized and in how these problems affected the people concerned. If gifted children have problems, then it is the scientist's job to identify them and find out what to do about them.

Social scientists also describe problems in terms of historical theory; they see present-day deviation from norms in terms of a past society. Thus, it might be claimed that there is more mental illness about than there used to be, usually with the addition of the current scapegoat that it's because of the 'strain of modern living'. There may indeed be more identified mental illness (of certain kinds), but this increase has probably nothing to do with 'modern stress' and everything to do with the extent of the facilities available to the mentally ill. In the days when they were generally ignored, while a relative few were incarcerated in prison-like conditions, the recorded number of mentally ill people was very low. When help is available, ill people come forward to be treated and registered and this is perhaps a key difference between a modern and a primitive state. Present-day totals of mentally ill people are often evaluated in relation to a concept of a past ideal society, which is never accurate and can be most misleading. For instance, when a national survey of 'lunatics' in England and Wales was carried out at the beginning of the last century, some counties were proud to reply that they contained none at all (Jones, 1972).

By statistical definition, gifted children are 'abnormal'; in everyday terms, there aren't many of them about – they form a tiny percentage of the whole population. The higher up the ability ranges a gifted child finds himself, the less statistically normal he is. To make this statement in relation to ability is acceptable, but how does this situation affect the behaviour of the individual concerned?

There is a theory, largely derived from Lemert (1951), that being different from the average can take two forms. The first is primary deviation in the form of biological differences like blindness, epilepsy or deformity, which can also be placed on a scale of normality. This scale would reflect how much is acceptable in a society and such thinking affects, for example, the treatment of handicapped children in relation to their education. It is only recently (DES, 1978a) that a proposal has been made in Britain to mingle most handicapped and normal children under one school roof. (Up to now the handicapped have been separated from normal children since they were first legally recognized in the British educational system.) This suggestion has engendered outraged cries from some educationalists, who feel that mixing children of very different abilities is detrimental to the education of the normal ones. There is undoubtedly a moral element in the accusations of 'educational tragedy' which fall on the reformers and it is the same morality which calls for gifted children to be separated into special schools, the less able being seen as dragging down the growth of more able children. Within this system, what may begin as rigid streaming within a school must logically conclude with more rigid segregation of certain children from others for reasons which are both moral and educational. The degree to which primary deviation is socially visible is a vital determinant of social reaction. Thus, minimal spasticity will not bar a child from mixing with his peers, but spasticity which causes ungainly movement will isolate the affected individual.

Secondary deviation arises from the first, when individuals behave as though they were deviant (Wing, 1978):

> 'But no matter what the original reasons for the deviations, they are not significant until they are organized subjectively into active roles, and become the social criteria for assigning status'.

Deviant individuals have to be aware of their own aberrations if they are to react to them and to fix them into their own life patterns. Deviations can remain primary, concerned only with specific symptoms and confined only to a given situation, as long as they are seen for what they are and dealt with in a socially acceptable way. When a person begins to use his primary deviance as a means of behaving differently, it becomes secondary deviance. He can use it as a means of defence – 'don't hurt me; I've got a bad leg' (a situation amusingly portrayed by Stephen Potter in *Lifemanship* (1950)) or of attack – 'I can say hurtful things to you because I am very old'. In this way an individual can indeed become the stereotype of society's reaction to him. Secondary deviation follows when the 'abnormal' person, as defined by society, adopts the appropriate way of life. These adaptations are in attitudes and behavioural changes of many kinds, but strong adaptive motives can turn a person with problems into a 'career' deviant. For instance, male homosexuals may adopt a 'camp' form of behaviour, which has no biological relationship with their sexual orientation, but is rather the product of social learning. A gifted child can learn to behave like a stereotype of a gifted child, with the accepted licence of difficult behaviour and entire approval from adults for it.

## Labelling.

A more general and easily acceptable theory than that of primary and secondary deviation is that of labelling. In this, the primary deviance is of so little matter that it can be disregarded; secondary considerations take over completely so that the label is the deviation. The label is a recognized description of a condition, but sometimes it is questionable whether the condition exists before the label is applied, or afterwards. For example, is there a problem with gifted children at all, or is their behaviour modified or even organized by the label which is so often hung on them? To be effective, a label need not be accepted or recognized by the affected individual so long as it is recognized by others.

Society has a set of stereotyped responses to violations of social norms. Gifted children must, by virtue of their tiny number, violate the social norm and are thus seen as 'deviant'. Labels such as 'frustrated', 'withdrawn', 'lonely', 'weedy' are stock responses. The evidence in Chapter 4 should undermine such a stereotype, but given the dynamics of human society and the emotional power of mythic thinking, it is unlikely to do so entirely. Problems which are recognized and defined must be seen in the social context in which they arose. It is comforting, in fact, when you have a problem, to find a label for it. People not only accept those that are given to them, but also seek out labels which can act as psychological crutches. For example, it is common to accept the description of 'victim of circumstance' which relieves the bearer of responsibility and saves effort. But a label is not a divine attribution, which has nothing to do with the recipient; it is ambiguous and negotiable. Labels can be accepted, rejected or exchanged.

Seeking out a label is an activity which can be seen and measured. People identify themselves by approaching organizations dedicated to the label of their choice. For example, when parents believe that their child has a reading problem they could take him to a Child Guidance Clinic, which may not offer them an acceptable label, or they could approach a Dyslexia Association, which might do so. The acquisition of a label may of itself provide sufficient satisfaction, but it can also serve as a launching pad for further action. Parents of children with problems usually have several possibilities of identification from which to choose, varying from the biological to the psychological. However, parents who seek help from an organization for gifted children believe, in the main, that they have a gifted child, though my research showed that this was not always the case.

Labelling can also victimize the recipient and is then a form of stigmatization; unfair labelling is the most unfortunate side-effect of any system of testing and selection. In Britain, children who did not go to a grammar school, as a result of being selected for another kind of education, often felt themselves to be labelled 'failures' for the rest of their lives. As this label seemed to be attached to about 75% of the population, it was perhaps not a very good thing for the nation's self-image. American children are tested every year of their school lives, as they go from grade to grade. These tests, which are supposed to identify both their achievement and potential, scatter diagnostic labels with impunity. In some achievement-motivated families, their children will be labelled as failures as a result of anything under an A grade in yearly examinations or of a less than perfect report from the school counsellor.

Even Alfred Binet, the originator of the intelligence test, recognized the problem in 1905 when he said that 'It would never be to one's credit to have attended a special school', meaning a school for less able pupils. There are inevitably mistakes in any test and all test material is explicit about its margin of error. School-age children are notably the most over-labelled group in the population and American research has found considerable evidence of a tendency to label by stereotypes (Mercer, 1975). She found that children of lower socio-economic class were assigned more 'retarded' labels, and that ethnic minority groups were mistakenly over-represented in schools for defective children. It follows that white children of high socio-economic status are more likely to be labelled gifted than other children. The effect of labelling is thus considerable, affecting both the child's self-concept and possibly her actual physical circumstances. The latter may result from putting her into a special school or class for children of her own labelled type. Whether this is a good, a bad or a false situation for the individual, it will certainly affect her whole life.

Jane Mercer, who made considerable discoveries about the way labels are given and their effects, has devised a new system of testing. Children in many American States are now compared in their test results with other children of the same socio-economic background. This is supposed to be fairer, but I believe that it would be even fairer if children were not labelled as being of any particular background before the testing begins, and even fairer again if the constant testing of American children were abolished or at least minimized. It is conceivable that getting rid of regular categorization activities and a stronger push towards child-centered education would allow each child to grow in her own time. Appropriate education would then lead towards her own fulfilment, but such a proposal could not be welcome to the many businesses which make profits from devising and marketing tests in the USA. However other countries manage well enough without this neat filing of their children; the only losers would be the test manufacturers.

The 'pluralistic' assessment of children, devised by Mercer, is already having an effect. A child who cannot do well on a conventional test of intelligence can now be measured on a new test and may emerge as 'gifted'. This, of course, is in comparison with a score for his own background, which has been predetermined by the tester. He should then enter a programme for gifted children, but in whose culture is the child now to be educated?

Labelling and its consequences are a matter of considerable moment in the world of social science and have engendered a wide range of research. There are many who hold that bad behaviour is caused by labelling, which itself arises from rules. These rules may be observable or unobservable, but breaking them is inevitably labelled as social deviance. The most obvious answer to this problem would be to get rid of the rules and the deviance should then go with them, but a society without rules is an impossibility. What we can do, though, is to minimize the rules. For example, many classroom rules are out of date and worthless; if they were dispensed with, there would not be any serious consequences. On the other hand, rules and labels can have positive effects in reducing deviant conduct and raising awareness of how that society works. Another possibility, especially effective with children, is to label the act rather than the child, i.e. to praise work rather than call the child gifted, with all its implications.

## The expectancy effect

Allied to the effects of labelling are those of expectancy, also known as the self-fulfilling prophecy. The influence of expectation on the part of parents and teachers has now entered the folklore of education through the work of Rosenthal and Jacobson (1968) mentioned earlier. Considerable attention has been given, particularly in places where teachers train, to the outcome of manipulating teachers' perceptions of their individual pupils. Education literature abounds with accounts of how pupils' performance is depressed or elevated by the way in which their teachers see them. If this phenomenon exists, there must be some means by which such information is passed between adult and child. It is the sort of effect which appears true on 'common-sense' grounds, but the evidence is stacked up against it. It is not known how teachers can differentiate between those children who are favourably and those who are unfavourably perceived in such a way that their classroom performance is affected.

McClelland (1961) uses the same idea to explain how, over the centuries, whole cultures have risen and fallen through their own expectations of themselves. When a culture is in the throes of psychological depression, down is the only way to go. Unfortunately, studies across cultures or periods of time are notoriously doubtful; for example, failure in one country might be success in another. A failed degree may be just that in the West, but on the Indian sub-continent, 'failed BA' signifies a certain standard of learning and therefore success, from which it may be possible to move on to a higher position in life. The expectancy effect can only be measured within well defined social limits. Though we have no entirely acceptable evidence for the effects of expectancy on the results of intelligence tests, there are examples of it in areas of social behaviour such as industry.

## The halo effect

This is a commonly used piece of psychological shorthand to indicate that increased attention to an individual increases his achievement. It is the most frequently offered explanation as to why children in any specialized education course do better than those in the general class. The argument is that increased attention to any child will improve that child's performance – no matter what is taught.

In the case of a gifted child, for instance, extra lessons on computer technology might be quite irrelevant to her general development as they stand, but their attention value is considerable and improved school performance can be attributed to this halo effect. On the other hand should this extra attention be given to all children, they would probably all improve in their school work: The argument seems to presuppose that not enough attention is given to individuals in the usual way of things, so that the extra is bound to have an effect. No doubt many educationalists would agree, but is it possible that enough attention could ever be paid to every child so that the halo effect could never be seen again?

## Social differences and abilities

In all societies there are behavioural differences between social groups which are all-pervading and can therefore be observed in the individual members of each group. In any aspect of the greater society, a relationship exists between the distribution of genetic characteristics on the one hand and social structures on the other. These social structures interact with the genetic components and in doing so tend to reinforce them. For example, the taboos on certain kinds of foods in some groups can inhibit the full growth of children, which is quite a different matter from an inability to obtain the food through lack of money. Assumptions of superiority in certain groups enable them to behave in ways which mean that they can take the best of what is available, without any need for a competitive struggle.

If these supporting social structures were to be hypothetically removed, there would be very little left to constitute identifiable innate differences between such groups as social classes. If, in addition, the variations within a social class which are attributable to individual differences were to be removed, there would be little if anything of significance remaining as direct differences between classes. Therefore, although we can reliably measure variations between the social classes for any moment in time, these differences are neither true for an individual nor constant for the class group.

Any number of individuals transplanted into another culture and class system will in time come to be like the people amongst them. The Jews who settled in China are a good example. In a country which was apparently unconcerned about these newcomers, they did eventually become assimilated and no longer exist as a definable group. In other countries, where there was an awareness of or an antipathy towards Jews, they retained their own culture. The physical differences between the Jews and the Chinese were obviously no barrier to assimilation, any more than colour differences are in some South American countries such as Venezuela or Cuba. There, especially in the cities, the people are of as mixed an origin as the world has to offer.

A family's life style and its consequent effects on parents' attitudes and on children's development are undoubtedly affected by the larger society outside, notably socio-economic class. There is a spectrum of differences in the way that children across the social classes are raised and it has been possible to measure these differences in Western societies. A number of longitudinal studies such as that of Douglas (1964), the work of the National Children's Bureau team under Kellmer Pringle (Davie, Butler and Goldstein, 1972) and research by the Newsons of Nottingham (1977) all support this view. The Plowden Report, *Children and Their Primary Schools,* included considerable discussion on the mechanisms leading to socio-economic class differences in ability test performances and educational achievement (DES, 1967, p. 349):

> 'Thus a result that 30 per cent of the school achievement was owing to (caused by) their parents' attitudes and 20 per cent to their parents' material circumstances, is a mere quantification of the view, which most sensible men would accept, that part must be owing to the one and part to the other.'

Although in general the evidence suggests that low socio-economic status is not the sole cause of variances in children's school progress or in behavioural deviances (Rutter, Tizard and Whitmore, 1970), low socio-economic status, as measured by a broad group of researchers, is associated with a lowering of IQ and with diminished educational attainment.

Hess and Shipman (1965) have studied for many years the effects of social class on child upbringing in Chicago. They conclude that:

> 'The working class environment produces a child who relates to authority rather than rationale; who although compliant, is not reflective in his behaviour; and for whom the consequences of an act are largely considered in terms of immediate punishment or reward, rather than future effects and long range goals.'

Other researchers (Tulkin and Kagan, 1972) have found class differences in mother–child interaction. Working class mothers did very much less listening and more often interrupted the baby when it was his turn to speak, but most importantly, they did not see the baby as a developing human being that they could assist in growing. They felt relatively powerless and did not aid and abet the child's development by stimulation and encouragement, as in the middle class way. This lowering of intellectual mothering has unfortunate effects on the baby's intellectual development. The evidence for this conclusion continues to accumulate from many studies, and may go some way towards explaining the over-representation of middle and upper class children in studies of the gifted.

Another problem that highly intellectual children may have to overcome in a family of poor cultural level is the lack of an adult model. A 'one-off' gifted child who cannot seek understanding or help from those responsible for his upbringing is in a very difficult position. She can either conform to her local social norms, and risk bitterness and unhappiness, or strike out in her own direction, which risks loss of the approval of her own family. Neither alternative is attractive.

## Intelligence

On the evidence available from studies of twins, brothers and sisters and foster children, it must be concluded that there is some genetic component in intelligence. Vernon (1955) recognized the genetic component of intelligence as that which is measurable by intelligence tests. But the active intelligence which works everyday and is based on the genetic component may not be entirely measurable; this is an amalgam of adaptations and modifications in intellectual behaviour which children learn as they grow. The relationship between the genetic and the learned aspects of intelligence is very complex and we do not know exactly what is involved. But in Halsey's words (1977):

'The growth of intelligence is dependent upon stimulation in social interaction, the use of language and the manipulation of objects.'

Piaget too, amongst others, sees the growth of intelligence as a complex restructuring of reflexes, leading on to the development and reforming of concepts which in turn develop into adult reasoning. But again this is dependent on the availability of experience.

Halsey distinguishes performance in intelligence tests as a particular kind of intelligence. He believes this to be only a sample of what is potentially measurable and, even so, the sample is biased because tests are specifically designed to predict educational success. Consequently, they only pick up the relevant aspects of intelligence, and in this way are reliable and do their stated jobs well. Thus, children who do well on intelligence tests *should* be expected to have an educationally supportive background and this most often proves to be the case.

We know that the two kinds of intelligence – the everyday one and the one that intelligence tests sample – each have a social component. If a child grows up without appropriate social stimulation, he will suffer in those aspects of intelligence. The biggest cause of genetic variation is not the individual concerned, but the population from which she comes. People who are recognizable as a group of similar general make-up are described as a gene pool.

There are limits to the variations found amongst children who may be born into a particular gene pool, which will vary according to four influencing factors: genetic drift, mutation, selection and migration. Gifted children can only be a relative phenomenon in terms of their gene pool since it is not possible to compare individuals for giftedness with the whole world, but only with their own population. Even within that group, members will vary; for example, some will be more fertile and will reproduce more than others. Each population has its own customs and rules of marriage which have their effects on future generations.

The reasons which make people change country, culture or class are primarily affected by the freedom people have to move at will and by the conditions they leave behind. But it is also probable that the new area will be selective as to who it takes in. Immigrants may be selected, as they were in the early part of this century for entry to the USA, on grounds of health and psychological acceptibility (Kamin, 1974). They are not then necessarily representative of the country they come from, or of their own gene pool, but of their acceptability to the host country. This is also true for people who change social class, either up or down; for instance physically attractive females are more likely to marry men of relatively higher status than themselves.

Using our present system of measurement, it is clear from many pieces of research that there is a far higher proportion of intellectually gifted children in the higher socio-economic classes than in the lower ones. Accepting the situation as it is does not imply a genetically ordained division between the classes, nor does it demonstrate that social cultures and environments produce different levels of intelligence. Either or both are possible causes of the differences.

The question of the relative distribution of gifted children among different cultures or social classes is largely a matter of social mobility and genetic migration. The relative numbers of such children appear to have remained stable over half a century, since Binet first began testing intelligence. Therefore, it can only be assumed that the families with such children who drop out of their social position are replaced by a similar number of those who come in. Increasing social mobility over this last century does not appear to have made any real difference to the balance of high ability children in different social groups.

Research evidence shows a direct relationship between fathers' occupational status and children's intelligence and my own results were no exception to this unvarying evidence.

With present social mobility and techniques of measurement, the problem for people concerned with the welfare of children is one of identifying the environmental components of social class which are of the greatest value for intellectual development.

## Verbal ability

The most striking and probably the most effectively measured difference between families of different socio-economic groups is in verbal interaction. As with any kind of stimulation, though, the quality is always more important than the quantity. In the transmission of language from one generation to the next, a fundamental kind of socialization is taking place. The child is not taught merely how to use language to express his ideas, but learns in this process how to think. It is probable (Sapir, 1929) that:

'we see and hear and otherwise experience very largely as we do because the language habits of our community predispose certain choices of interpretation'.

It follows that limited language acquisition also limits thoughts and ideas and, by the same token, the greater the variety of language, the wider intellectual development will be. But the style of intellectual activity is directed by the language that children learn.

There is no need to look for any indirect influence of language on thought; speech is the obvious and immediately available behaviour by which language can be related to culture. Thus, an important part of 'black' American cultural behaviour is to speak in 'Black English'. Terman (1972) has illustrated the way in which it functions

'both as an expression of imposed pariah status and as a complex representation of a cultural system which not only mirrors the former, but serves as a refuge from it'.

Although its methodology was questionable, Bernstein's research (1972) was the first to point out the linguistic differences between social classes and their effects on school achievement. However, he was not alone in finding that middle class mothers are more explicit, convey more information when they speak, and talk more to their children when they play with them than working class mothers. This verbal interaction is both informative and educational to the children (Wooton, 1974; Clark, 1976). Middle class mothers also spend considerably more time than working class mothers on the equally important activity of listening to their children and responding in conversational style to what has been said. Many studies of the use of language in children have found that both the topic and the listener are essential influences on the amount and complexity of children's spoken language. However, Margaret Clark, in her study of very early readers (1976), cautions:

'that it is crucial to explore the parents' perceptions of education and the support and experiences they provide by measures far more sensitive and penetrating than social class, father's occupation - or even education of parents'.

She found that it was in homes where books were an integral part of the contents and where there were plenty of rich, stimulating experiences that children became early readers, irrespective of social class.

In Manchester, Wiseman (1964) found that the number of books available in the home was positively related to a child's reading attainment. In a highly literate home, a child will almost certainly be read to, as well as talked to, and no matter how gifted, a child still has to learn to read. From the very beginning, a gifted child benefits greatly from instant assistance by an adult who can supply any word which is not understood from the context. Children will obviously progress better if there is someone around who can give this instant encouragement, as well as playing with them, even at the expense of whatever else they were doing.

## Other abilities

Children can obviously be gifted in many respects other than intelligence. It was far from being my intention at the outset of my research to concentrate on the intellectually gifted, but, in fact, the group of people who had joined the National Association for Gifted Children had, in all but four out of 70 cases, joined because of their child's supposed intellectual gifts. As these parents and their children formed the basis of my sample, the research was obliged to concern itself with their stated interests, rather than with the general situation of gifted children. The other four children were believed to be gifted musicians and all attended a selective school for musical children in Manchester, where the fine selection procedure in itself validated the parents' belief in their children. My own earlier research on children who were gifted (or talented) in music and fine art provided evidence about the environments of such children, as well as the basis for the research being presented here (Freeman, 1976b and 1977).

In this first study, children who were outstanding in either music or fine art were searched out in the industrial city of Salford. They were children who were attending normal city schools and who had not previously been identified, nor given special education as being talented. They were matched for age, sex and school class to provide a control group of children who were not aesthetically talented and all the children, their homes and their schools were investigated. The research was concerned with differences that might be found between these talented children and their controls, with respect to the environmental influences that operated on the achievements of all the children.

Analysis of the results showed clearly that those children who had been chosen as aesthetically outstanding scored significantly more highly in the memory and perception tests in music and fine art than their controls. The environments of these talented groups of children also proved to be heavily biased, appropriately, either in the music or the fine art direction. Both the talented and control children had had access to musical instruments and art materials, as well as to extra lessons, provided free of charge by the local education authority. Both school and home had managed to provoke interest, but it was only the children from homes where music or art was given priority who were identified as talented.

There was, however, an overlap of ability between these two types of aesthetically talented children. From the evidence gathered, it was possible to say that, had either group of specifically talented children been exposed to the upbringing of the other, then they might well have exchanged their fields of expertise. By the same reasoning, had the non-talented control children been brought up in either the musical or artistic families, their abilities would have been, at the very least, considerably improved. The unavoidable conclusion was that parental attitudes and provision were of essential importance in the development of aesthetic perception and practice in those children.

Physically gifted children arise from a similar family situation. In its most practical aspects, family encouragement and help are vital for the continuous extra practices, which usually have to take place in the most unsocial hours. Particular cultures, such as the Soviet Union and Australia, produce a disproportionate number of physically gifted children. Unless the state takes over the financial support of these children, the extra coaching required would price all but the richest parents out of the competition. The one exception to this rule is probably boxing, which has always been regarded as the poor boy's way to accepted status. But again, the boy needs financing and is usually taken under the wing of a boxing gymnasium as a protégé. Ballet dancers have the same problems and normally have to win scholarships to specific institutions in order to obtain further coaching. It is rare for a dancer to emerge from a background which has not been encouraging.

Giftedness in children must be as varied as are abilities. Moral and financial support is essential for the development of all gifts which are distinctly above those of other children. But what is a gift in one culture is disregarded in another, so that support will vary with what is considered to be valuable.

# CHAPTER 3

# Judging Giftedness

---

Giftedness is only at one extreme of a considerable range of childhood behaviours. Along the spectra of these behaviours, there are qualitative change-points, i.e. levels at which a change can be seen, like that between water and steam. The specialist tends to see mainly the more severe end of any spectrum, yet a child can only be understood in terms of what is normal. Being labelled gifted does imply that it is a condition which, if unclear, can yet be recognized. One of the difficulties in measuring abilities is the considerable haziness of their change-points – if these exist at all. To be gifted must also be to overlap and synthesize with other children in many respects. A child must be regarded primarily as a child and any special abilities then taken into consideration only as part of the whole growing person. It is not scientifically acceptable to diagnose a child as gifted and then to explain the rest of him from that vantage point; that is, assume that a child shall behave in a special way and be treated in a special way because he is labelled gifted. It must be the other way round. A child is a child first with special abilities or special problems second.

The psychologist does not think she has said all there is to be said about a child when the conclusion is reached that he is gifted. A theory has then been put forward that can be tested in various ways, but it would be a poor psychologist who did not use a wide variety of other skills, including those social skills which she has developed in common with other mature human beings.

# PHYSICAL DEVELOPMENT

The rate and extent of physical growth varies greatly between different children and these natural differences are relatively little affected by environmental factors. But it is most important that people such as parents, teachers or doctors who live and work with children should recognize that these differences do exist and should be alert to the various effects and problems that they create.

There have been many attempts to describe growth in terms of neat mathematical curves, but these have all been unsuccessful. The main problem is in deciding how it should be measured; for example, length and width are but two of the many aspects of muscle growth. An individual's growth can only be measured in relation to his own personal pattern. As with mental development, averages of physical growth, taken cross-sectionally from an age-group of children, become flattened and distorted and therefore doubtful as a means of comparison between individuals. The peaks of the individual growth spurts are thus smoothed into one apparent continuum. In life, these spurts can be seen as brief active changes in the rate of growth. However, imperfect though they are, we still have to use averages as measures by which we can judge whether children are growing-normally, so that something can be done about it if they're not. The most accurate method of measuring growth is to divide it into aspects to be measured, since different parts of the body and tissues grow at different rates. For example, the brain, together with the skull covering it and the eyes and ears, develops earlier than any other part of the body and consequently has its own characteristic growth curve.

## Development before birth

Even today, it is difficult to find out exactly what influences an unborn baby's development. We have X-rays, and all sorts of investigatory techniques, but still a good deal of knowledge comes from babies who leave the uterus unexpectedly early. Tragic accidents, such as that of the drug thalidomide, pinpointed precisely which cells are developing at what time by preventing their normal development. German measles in the mother affects the eyes of the unborn baby only between the first and twelfth week of pregnancy. After that, there is no altered development due to this disease. In this way, we know that weeks 1–12 are the vulnerable ones for eyes. Such a time may also be called a critical or sensitive period.

Before birth, the baby is being formed so that cells are dividing, redividing and forming body structures. Studies at Columbia University (Winick, 1971) have shown that severe malnutrition, if it happens at a stage in development when the cells should be dividing, may inhibit this division. The more rapid the rate of cell division at the time of starvation, the more damaging the effect. The division of cells does not stop and wait for better times, though cell growth does.

A study on the long-term effect of undernutrition before birth was made by Stein *et al.* (1975). They looked at the effects of severe wartime famine in three Dutch cities. In particular, they investigated the effects on the boys, who were born in that time, as they later entered compulsory military service. They found that men who had been undernourished before they were born were not different in height, weight or mental ability from those who had been adequately nourished. Nor were there effects to be found as to family size, social class and birth order. They concluded that prenatal nutrition by itself could not alter potential mental competence, but that if it were combined with malnutrition in infancy, it did affect mental ability.

There is in biology a 'catch-up' mechanism, by which an animal which has deviated from its individual growth course can still return to the original path, if conditions change. A child can be seen to catch up in this way, after a long illness, provided he is well fed and looked after. But undernutrition in a child's very early life is another matter and this more serious effect is probably concerned with the time of cell division.

Birthweight has a very close relationship with the later ability levels of children, as seen on testing. Probably the most pertinent aspect in relation to a child's future possibility of giftedness is the kind of nutritional background he comes from. Poor environmental circumstances, especially of food for the mother, result in babies having a lowered birthweight. A considerable proportion of underweight babies fail to develop the same levels of mental ability as normal children.

This feature can pass through two generations or more (Tanner, 1978):

'Mothers who, because of adverse circumstances in their own childhood, have not achieved their full growth potential may produce smaller foetuses than they would have done had they grown up under better conditions.'

There is no doubt that this matter of physical environment is of essential importance for a child's intellectual development. The likelihood of a gifted child coming from a barely nourished family must therefore be slight. This is the beginning of the great divide between children who will achieve their potential and those who will not. The effects of a poor environment, such as deprivation in an industrial city or a sudden famine in an underdeveloped country, take a lot of repair facilities, which are not normally available. It is not possible to push up a child's ability by extra feeding, but good food does provide the essential fuel for physical and mental growth.

New born babies differ not only in behaviour, but in size and shape. Tanner (1974) points out that variation amongst infants is as great as it is among children and adults. Variation in physiological maturity is large 'amounting to about 3 or 4 weeks of development among babies all of exactly 40 weeks' gestational age'. He suggests that it would be strange if the effects of these variations were to be negligible. But in spite of these differences between children at the time of their birth, brain development continues unabated from conception. Neurological development is unaffected by the normal passage of the baby from uterus to the outside world, though of course it can be hampered by an abnormal birth. For example, there is no relationship between the onset of conditioned reflexes and birth date; the conditioned reflex is related in time to the baby's conception and not to the time of its birth.

## Boys and girls

The singular and most obvious difference between boy and girl babies at birth is in their genital structure. Barring accidents of development, the internal and external genitalia are always either male or female. Other physical sex differences which exist are matters of varying proportion between the sexes rather than of a different design. The sex hormones, which initiate and control sexual differences, are controlled by the brain, i.e. the hypothalamus. Thus there is at least one aspect of brain functioning which is different in boys and girls, and which might possibly be affected by altered circumstances during critical periods.

Girls grow up faster than boys and the difference can be seen even before birth. At birth, girls are about four to six weeks physically more mature than boys; by puberty, the difference corresponds to two years' development. This is possibly the reason why more girls than boys survive at birth. It is certainly the reason why girls do better at school in late puberty. Boys are a little taller than girls from birth to adolescence; then girls take the lead for a while until boys overtake them entirely in young adulthood.

Each child has his or her own maturation rates, which are predictable at birth. They become particularly noticeable at puberty when perfectly normal children can find themselves either well beyond or else lagging behind their friends in development. It seems that heredity plays a large part in deciding the individual 'tempo of growth'. We need, but do not possess, a measure of developmental age or physiological maturity, which would represent an individual more faithfully than chronological age. The education of children would be much improved by the availability of such a measure. However, there are guidelines, recognizable as stages of growth, such as loss of baby teeth or the beginnings of puberty, and skeletal maturity can be measured by X-ray techniques.

## Physical development and mental ability

There is a curious relationship between height and mental ability. University students are always the tallest people in the country, while educationally subnormal children are smaller than normal children, even when their fathers' socio-economic level is taken into consideration. Height and mental capability are both affected by stress, growth hormone being inhibited under stressful conditions. Height, intelligence and school achievement levels are higher in urban than in rural children.

There is evidence that an individual's physical growth tempo is related to his or her mental growth. Children who are physically more advanced than others of the same chronological age score more highly in tests of mental ability. This difference is consistent across ages, so that children with a faster growth tempo always have a better chance of doing well in age-linked tests, such as end-of-term class exams. Even on the straightforward measure of height, as one aspect of growth, the Stanford–Binet IQ score is increased by 0.67 points for each centimetre of stature, or $1\frac{1}{2}$ IQ points per inch (Tanner, 1978). Children of large families tend to be shorter than children of small families; they also do less well in IQ tests. But of course, all the socio-environmental circumstances have to be taken into consideration for each child. It is now clear that some of this relationship between children's height and IQ continues into adult life.

There is a difference in height between the children of managerial and unskilled workers; the higher status children are taller. The National Child Development Study (Goldstein, 1971) in its survey of all British children found an overall difference of 3.3 cm between the seven-year-old children of managerial and of unskilled fathers. Some of this was due to the faster tempo of growth in the well off, but much of the difference will continue into adult life. This relationship of occupational class to height, which is found all over the world, has now eased off in the more economically egalitarian countries such as Sweden. From this, it could be expected that there will be less overall variation in intelligence within the population of such countries.

The emotional response of children to their physical growth must be considerable. When their growth, though normal, is not in step with that of their contemporaries, children's self-images may be damaged. Boys seem to suffer more from these comparisons than girls, especially at puberty. Physical prowess is valued by Western society as an aspect of manliness – the body is very much a representative of the person. Consequently, the muscular, athletic boy tends to dominate his fellows before puberty; then, even though the others catch up, he can often hold on to his early lead. Unfortunately for him, the unathletic, lanky boy tends to get pushed further and further into a position of low status as adolescence progresses.

Late developing girls suffer too. They may be teased about their obviously flat chests and so perceive themselves as not properly female. But early maturing girls may be embarrassed and take on the familiar adolescent stoop to hide their new breasts; for both girls and boys, early maturation means the need for a longer control of the growing sex drive.

Research (Mussen and Jones, 1957) has shown that early or late physical development in boys can be associated with significant changes in their personalities; outstanding leaders tend to come from the early maturing group. Later maturers were less self confident and were less easy to get on with. In adult life too, the early maturing boys became more sociable and less neurotic than the late maturing boys. However, the latter appear to be more sensitive and understanding.

We do not inherit height, nor ability; we inherit their genetic structure. The genes affect the development of the foetus, which at the same time is interacting with its uterine environment. After birth, the development of the child is affected by its new, even more complex and changing environment.

Some interactions are of vital importance, such as those which occur during 'sensitive' or critical periods. These times have been found to be significant in the physical development of children, but we are less sure of their relationship to mental development. There is a strong possibility, however, that they may be effective in the promotion of specific talents. Playing a musical instrument to the level of giftedness may well depend on opportunity at a sensitive stage. There is a recognized uncertainty as to how the two function together.

As an example of a physical critical period, there is a condition which is called a 'lazy eye' where one of a child's eyes becomes dominant, sometimes to such an extent that the other ceases to function. If a blind is put over the good eye, the lazy one starts to be used again. However, if the condition is not noticed in time, by about the age of five, the child never develops proper binocular vision. The genes have been effective in bringing the development of the eyes to the point where they should be used, but if they are not, then permanent damage occurs. The experience of continued binocular seeing is essential during this critical period of retinal cell development. Animal experiments have demonstrated the existence of this critical period in their mental development and there is some hotly contested evidence to show that it exists in human development. But generalizing from animals to humans or from physical to mental development is questionable. We can, however, say that good steady stimulation promotes continued intellectual development, whereas a deficiency of it is detrimental to a child.

## Health

There is an undoubted relationship between physical and mental health, which has been scientifically verified over and over again. Some illnesses such as asthma, eczema and hay fever can be primarily reactions to stress, as well as to allergic stimuli (Davie *et al.* 1972; Illingworth, 1964). Illingworth, the paediatrician, has in fact stated that many of the children who suffer from eczema 'are mentally above average', although he did not say that they were likely to be gifted. He also suggested that children from the higher social classes are more predisposed to allergic reactions than those from the lower classes.

A small but fascinating study was conducted by Meyer and Haggerty (1962) in the USA of sore throats in children of fifteen middle class families. Every two or three weeks for a year, the investigators made a throat culture from each of the children. Using both diaries kept by the mothers and interviews, they noted all the disruptive events in each family's life during this period. All their measures of infection, with or without signs of illness, were four times more likely to happen after a distressing event, such as the child witnessing a road accident. But they were also more likely in the context of 'chronic family stress' and it was concluded that emotional and physical factors combined in some way to produce this type of illness.

Generally speaking, the internal organs of the human body function smoothly and efficiently so that their owner is virtually unaware of their existence. Only when there is some form of physical distress is the brain conscious of the sensation of what is going on internally. The time when this kind of disorder is most likely to happen is one of emotional disturbance, when the person is frightened, nervous or angry. The nature and degree of this functional disorder depends on the individual's constitution and sensitivity, as does the extent to which he is aware of what is happening. Respiratory disorders such as asthma nearly always follow some sort of emotional disturbance; even the fear of asthma itself can actually bring on attacks. Stomach complaints in children too are associated with stress; they seldom cause waking from sleep and are usually the result of nervous intestinal spasm.

Awareness of or sensitivity to the bodily state produces fear, anxiety and resentment; it is a vicious circle which may either cause or increase the functional disorder itself. What first set this circle in motion may be a real and palpable source of fear, or else a disease which disturbs the body's function. But once it has been set up, it can become self-perpetuating and remain long after the original cause has ceased to operate. Some children have a mental and physical constitution of such a type that this vicious circle is more easily set up. Their internal organs readily suffer malfunction, they are intensely aware both of their bodies and surroundings and they are emotional people who are an easy prey to fear. They often happen to be highly intelligent, but unless they can be given a proper understanding of and insight into their troubles, this intelligence is no help to them.

Owing to the nature of their training, most doctors attend to the disordered function itself and there are many drugs which may be used to bring the delinquent organ under control. Some, such as tranquilizers and sedatives, may also be used to reduce the level of awareness, calming people's emotions so that these are less overwhelming. This awareness of symptoms is also greatly diminished by activities in which the person concerned can be deeply involved and so less aware of his body functions.

Failure to deal with the fear will generally result in failure to cure, but, with children, it is the fears of the parents which are often the most important. The parents are so close to the child that their emotional state is easily conveyed to her. Physical symptoms are not necessarily an indication of bodily abnormality and though worry and fear are part and parcel of life, they need not become dominant. Periods of stress are bound to occur in the life of any child and it is at these times that functional disorders are likely to be most troublesome. By far the commonest causes of them are family upsets and school difficulties.

The primary source of advice for parents who have a child with a physical functional disorder is examination by a doctor to see whether disease is present. Should the doctor fail to find any organic abnormality in the child, there is a possibility that parents may dismiss him as incompetent or disbelieving of their problems. In such a situation, the parents' fear or resentment is increased. But an aware doctor can show parents by careful and attentive listening and examination of the child that they are believed and that there is no reason to be afraid. On the basis of medical reassurance, the doctor is able to recommend other helping agencies such as psychologists and counsellors who may be able to assist the parents to see their problem in better perspective and, in doing so, relieve the symptoms of distress.

## ASSESSING ABILITIES

Abilities are difficult to define, being concepts without a material existence. It is only by observing children's actual behaviour that we can infer the presence of some intangible entity and try to measure it. However, there is always the danger that this measured inference becomes seen, to all intents and purposes, as the ability itself.

Intelligence tests measure behaviour that psychologists infer from the concept of intelligence – not the ability itself. Hence the somewhat trite definition of intelligence as that which intelligence tests measure. Different intelligence tests produce different results and the overlap between them varies greatly. Consequently, they must to some extent be measuring different aspects of intelligence or even other aspects of the process of answering tests. This state of affairs had led to the formation of a number of models of intelligence, made up of a variety of different abilities with varying degrees of inter-relationship.

Aesthetic abilities are an area in which performance and understanding are perceptibly not the same thing. Music and fine art are fraught with questions about the meaning of musicality and of being artistic. The appreciation and practice of an art appear to be different, if overlapping, abilities. Both are open to cultural influences, but particularly appreciation since it is free of the ties of technical skill.

Learning to practise painting or music is very dependent on what is available in a child's environment. Involvement in aesthetics is probably more affected by chance than any other subject. There may be very many children of great ability who, because of poor environmental circumstances, both of provision and disapproval, will hardly brush with aesthetics. Other children may acquire prodigious instrumental technique as a skill, without commitment or understanding of the art. In an earlier piece of research, I found that social factors were highly relevant to observable aesthetic talent (Freeman, 1977). With many children, the lasting commitment to aesthetics seems to come about in early adolescence whereas childhood enthusiasm does not always last.

Though most tests of musical ability attempt to measure dimensions of musical aptitude, such as rhythm or pitch, there is a counter-argument that musical ability is unitary and cannot be split into parts, so that bits of it could be measured separately. Tests of fine art ability lag far behind those for music and the few that exist cannot be used with confidence. Such ability has to be judged by 'experts' and is thus a matter of subjective opinion. The assessment of musical ability too, even when formal tests are used, is rounded off with an audition to 'experts'. Children gifted in fine art are constantly concerned with visual presentation, attempting to record the images they see. Their presentations are illuminating and revealing; they bear the imprint of the artist, both in emphasis and in relationships between colours or shapes. As well as mastery of the techniques of using their materials, they are sensitive to their aesthetic qualities; this is not the same as learned competence. Fine artists are hard workers who go on and on with a project until it is acceptable. Some aspects of fine art call for a high degree of intelligence while others require an intuitive emotional ability, but tuition which emphasises skill over imagination can be very detrimental to gifted children. They need time, recognition and encouragement above all else.

Giftedness in English takes many forms. Such children show an unusually sensitive response to literature, a mature and sustained capacity to analyse and express the text and their responses. Gifted infants take a particular delight in playing with words and may speak very early. Both written and oral English gifts have the power to affect the recipients emotionally, but these two aspects of giftedness in English are not given equal weight in schools. Creativity with words is sometimes sacrificed to the techniques of officially accepted grammar. The recognition of giftedness in English is very susceptible to the ideas of the English teacher in school and gifted writers of many kinds were not seen to be outstanding at English in their school years. It is a facility which spills over into many walks of life and is directly related to the way we measure intelligence – the mainspring of all mental activity.

Foreign language ability is not necessarily related directly to skill at reading and writing in one's own language. Gifted language speakers require a high degree of mimicking ability, while, for others, their command of the written word far exceeds their oral abilities. It is possible that the reading and talking aspects of languages are a feature of general intellectual ability, as I found in my research (p. 178). The gifted linguist needs verbal and mimicking skills as well as an empathy for the language. Whereas a highly intelligent, hard working child can master the technique of a foreign language, the gifted linguist has the facility to 'become' it for a while, using its words and phrases like a native speaker.

Giftedness can be seen in many forms of movement, both individual (such as dance and swimming) and in competitive sports. Opportunity is again influential in enabling potentially gifted athletes to develop their abilities. There are undoubtedly many physically able children who, for want of facilities and encouragement, will never emerge as gifted. The 'experts', i.e. experienced physical education teachers, will readily spot individual attributes of strength endurance, agility and co-ordination, but all this is dependent on seeing a child in action. But the other necessary attributes of physical giftedness such as interest, determination and the capacity to learn cannot be prejudged. As with other abilities, if a school has a dedicated and enthusiastic teacher on its staff, more gifted children will emerge from there. Chance is always active and the proportion of physically gifted children in a school is unlikely to be attributable to its catchment area. Competitive sport is particularly affected by cultural moves; games are promoted to varying extents in different parts of the world. Boys particularly may be taken up because of their gifts by the society around them. But such is the general support for children gifted at competitive sport in England that no parent, to my knowledge, sought membership of the National Association for Gifted Children on behalf of their gifted footballer or athlete.

Mathematical gifts are identifiable at an early age. Infants playing with bricks or patterns can be distinguished from potential artists by their ability to discuss the various possibilities of their ideas. The ability to calculate comes later though and verbal ability is closely tied to mathematical ability. Gifted mathematicians may reveal themselves by 'the original remark, the unexpected question, the leap to the abstract, the distrust of intuition, a persistence and a desire for perfection. They may detect ambiguity or imprecision in the teacher's mathematical language' (DES, 1977).

Children who are very able at mathematics are more likely to be streamed, promoted or given special provision in school than other gifted children. This is probably essential in formal classroom teaching where individual gifts for investigation and unusual responses to mathematical problems would be unacceptable. But where work is not 'set' and the teacher is understanding, there will be room for the gifted to manoeuvre. As with other types of gifts, rapid acceleration in mathematics, well beyond the child's age group, runs the risk of future boredom and loss of interest. The child cannot go on to further mathematics because this would involve moving to another educational establishment and she is still in need of the rest of her education. Being top of a secondary school in mathematics at the age of 14 often implies a long time treading water in what should be an exciting subject. Mathematical gifts come to the young and flower in youth; they are of particular importance to educationalists concerned with gifted children.

It may be seen that the perception of gifts in children is very dependent on social and cultural factors. Chance, in the form of opportunity and encouragement, is often vital. The sensitivity of adults around is important to the development of a child's abilities, but of course each adult's own personality and expectations will affect his perception of the child. All teachers must be aware of the untapped potential which passes before them daily, but no child can ever realize all his abilities to the full; life is not long enough. What we can do, by means of improved assessment, is to recognize those gifts which *have* opportunities to develop in the child's social environment.

## Judging potential

There is an obvious similarity between judging potential and fortune telling, but it can be said for psychology that it is more scientific.

Parents and teachers do judge children's potential in a variety of personal, subjective and very inefficient ways. Certainly, the best predictor of future achievement is past achievement, but that gives no idea of untapped ability or aptitude. An aptitude for a subject may not show itself until a child is well into a learning situation. Though that is rather an expensive way to find potential, it may be the only way. For that reason alone, an all-round education is essential for the growth of differing abilities. A good aptitude test could result in more effective instruction, but they are still few and far between.

As yet, the long-term prediction of the development of individual ability is still a little hazy, though in group terms it is rather better. Judging the probability of growth in abilities is based on accumulated evidence of achievement from many children, as well as the knowledge of how they have progressed from there. It is only on this evidence of the past performances of large numbers of children that predictions for individuals can be made. It is assumed in such predictions that pupils have all had the same educational experiences and opportunities. When this is not so, the interpretation of an individual's score will be misleading, unless such factors are taken into account.

Effective prediction of educational potential would, of course, be highly beneficial to children; as a basis of intervention, it could be used to encourage the predicted outcome, thus making it more certain. But it could also be used to avert predicted problems from handicapping conditions. Good prediction is essential in deciding the relative merits of different types of education and psychological programmes. Without good prediction, the reaction to a situation is just a shot in the dark.

During the first quarter of this century, the overwhelming influence in psychology was a belief that human characteristics, whether of hereditary or environmental origin, were fixed from a very early age. This idea, based on little more than guesswork in its time, is still with us today. On this assumption, prediction was relatively straightforward; measure a young child and you will know how she will progress. Added to this, the effect of social expectations arising from childhood environmental conditions would serve to reinforce predictions. But this circle is so often broken that it makes the idea of fixed ability in childhood more than doubtful.

Traditionally, intelligence tests measure innate capacity and can be used to measure potential, at least of scholastic achievement, though, of course, this depends on what is required as evidence of scholastic achievement. Jensen (1973a) suggested that 60% of all the differences in school achievement are accounted for by individual differences in intelligence. There is undoubtedly a relationship between achievement and intelligence. But it is questionable whether intelligence is the cause of school success or whether the reverse holds true – that scholastic success itself brings about an increase in intelligence test scores.

In a broad sense, the IQ score is an excellent predictor of worldly success. Twenty-five years after their selection, the subjects of Terman's study of children with an IQ of over 140 gave impressive evidence of the predictive value of their IQs. By then, 71% of the sample were in high-status professional and managerial occupations, compared with 13.8% of the Californian population as a whole. Their average income was higher than that of the typical college graduate (Terman and Oden, 1959; Oden, 1968). In these terms, IQ can predict the level of achievement for decades. But it must be remembered that Terman's sample population had a clear head-start over other children because of their home backgrounds. Advantages in intelligence scores can, however, be revised even late in adolescence. Clarke and Clarke (1976) have rounded up considerable evidence to show that children who have been deprived in their early lives and who have done badly on measures of ability have shown great improvement under improved conditions. When the children received mental and physical nurturing, they seemed to return to their probably original level of potential ability. This was at ages much older than was considered possible until recently; even adolescents were able to gain considerably. In general, the so-called inherent differences in ability are being regarded as dominant very much less than they were even a few years ago.

Using the results of intelligence tests as a basis for the identification of potential giftedness involves some recognized disadvantages. The question of test accuracy for children of different environments is troublesome, as is the relative impact of heredity and environment on test performance. Test differences between groups of children from abundant and deprived environments have been found in most studies. It would be expected that environments which encourage the development of language would stimulate the development of general intelligence. The effect of a favourable environment may also explain how greater proportions of the gifted come from better educated parents and more affluent homes than the average. This has been found to be true for minority groups as well as for the general population. However, the assumption of the paucity of gifted children among the poorer sections of society is in itself distorting. It can affect the selection of gifted children by researchers, to the detriment of the children concerned.

Early recognized gifted children do seem to preserve their high test scores into high adolescence or early adulthood. But gifted girls are more likely to regress to the average of the general (American) college population than boys (Miles, 1954). This could be due to the differences in the development rates of boys and girls. If girls are measured in late childhood, at about 7–10 years old, they are normally found to be physically and mentally more advanced than boys of the same age. During adolescence, the boys catch up and so the relative proportions of their measurement results are altered. This early maturing of girls is also the probable cause of their being more likely than boys to be chosen by teachers as being gifted.

## Very early learning experience

The belief that early social experience is supremely effective throughout an individual's life is reflected in the whole history of Western thinking. Freud considered the first six years to be the essential time for the formation of neuroses, while the teaching order of Jesuits considered that they needed four years to organize an infant into their ways of thought. The saying 'the child is father to the man' sums it up for the English-speaking world.

The corollary of this view is that the effect of later experience is very much less significant. A practical example of this way of thinking in America was in the vast resources poured into the Head Start programme, compared with, say, the resources available to adolescents with learning difficulties. But in Britain, although there is considerable public demand for nursery school places, the resources are being used at present for older children through the raising of the school leaving age from 15 to 16 years.

However, evidence is beginning to show that very early experience does not hold the key to the whole of a child's future development. Learning experiences are not normally of a one-off nature; they tend to be repeated many times, although isolated instances can undoubtedly be effective. Experience is a continuous process for most children and what is missed the first time round will come again. But there can be no reinforcement of a learning procedure if it is not repeated. Belief in the supreme effectiveness of early experience is an example of almost total acceptance of environment as the shaper of people – an acceptance which has been shared by people whose views are otherwise very divergent.

Ann and A.D.B. Clarke (1976) have presented a considerable volume of argument and evidence, including their own research, which concludes that the early years do not by themselves impose irreversible influences on later development. They outline the deficiencies in earlier evidence on this subject, taken from animals and deprived children.

The best known exponent of the supposed effects of early 'maternal deprivation' was John Bowlby (1951), presented in his monograph for the World Health Organization. In subsequent years, it affected the lives of all concerned parents, although less so today. He believed that the separation of mother and child, sometimes for quite short times, could lead to permanent distress in the child. A long-term 'mother substitute' was permissible, but not to be recommended. The effect of the report was mainly to produce intense feelings of guilt in mothers. But it also altered their behaviour; labouring under 'expert' opinion, they were now unable to leave their infants for any length of time, day or night, for several years. Bowlby helped to sensitize the public to the baby's needs, but he consistently overestimated the effects of early learning experiences.

The Bowlby thesis was based on research, both by himself and others. However, the concept of maternal deprivation was so broad as to be difficult to define and examine. It did not include the effects of different forms of mother–child separation, nor the extent of duration of the experience, nor what happened before and after deprivation. By the 1960s the validity of Bowlby's advice was becoming doubtful – and Rutter's *Maternal Deprivation Reassessed* (1972) presents the contemporary view. In this the baby is regarded increasingly as a dynamic being, who to some extent brings about her own learning experiences (see p. 39).

It is possibly the effects of early experience which act on later experiences to reinforce themselves, so that early learning is seen to be prolonged. Similar early and late behaviour may not then arise from the same early cause, but from later indirect causes, so that the child becomes the unwitting agent of her own later difficulties. It is essential to be aware of the events following learning experiences which may prolong what would otherwise be transistory effects, good or bad. For example, children who are hospitalized are often assumed to suffer because of that time of isolation from home. But Douglas (1975) has found that children in hospital are not typical of the general population. They tend to come from large families, with manual occupations and with parents who take little interest in their schooling. Early admission to hospital may be a symptom of present and future disadvantage, rather than the cause of adolescent disturbance.

The Clarkes' main conclusion is that early learning experience is relative, not absolute. It is:

'mainly important for its foundational character.
By itself and when unrepeated over time, it serves no more than a link in the

developmental chain, shaping proximate behaviour less and less powerfully as age increases.'

The whole of development is important, not merely the early years. As yet there is no evidence that any developmental stage is more important than others. In the long term they are all important.

If there are particular times when children give a brief, but intensive, response to the environment, one might expect early experience to have disproportionate effects on later development. But the idea of critical periods has not been shown to be as vital to humans as it is in the animal world. For example, Lenneberg (1967) sees the critical period for acquiring primary speech as lasting till puberty - a long span of criticalness.

Critical periods are supposed to be at their most sensitive during the early years of life, but they also affect the later years. If early learning were to be timed to coincide with critical periods, we could expect it to be particularly efficient and persistent. Unfortunately there is no scientific evidence for this. However, the Montessori method of infant education is based on the idea of teaching at such times as the child is open to learning. In order to do this, the teacher must be flexible and sensitive and be able to act when the child is ready.

The gifted child is often thought to be in particular need of early learning experiences. The myth of giftedness, as it stands at present, assumes that if the child is not given a rich environment, she will become frustrated and delinquent. In fact, the gifted infant, by virtue of her extra abilities, will be far more able to take advantage of whatever opportunities for learning may arise. A baby with an active mind and body is more likely to search out experience than one who lets life pass by. In this way, a gifted infant does indeed obtain early enrichment, but she also has a continuingly richer life.

Determination of a child's future does not stop when the early years are over. Human development is a gradual process of genetic and environmental interactions. It would be better to avoid the use of the term 'critical period', with its implication of specific times for learning and its overtones of zoology. Instead, the gentler term of sensitivities would be more in keeping with human child development; this has implications of awareness and openness to learning which wax and wane in relation to different processes at different times. To change a word is to change concept and, in this case, it also means changing a whole way of looking at childhood.

## Assessing achievement

Gifted children are probably most recognizable in the area of achievement. The assessment of achievement, however, can only be the assessment of performance, which is how well a child does at a certain task. But the term achievement implies a wide variety of performance behaviours, having different meanings for different people. When a mark is given to a standard of excellence, whose excellence is being used? McClelland (1961) proposed that achievement in the individual is related to the prevailing cultural values. But within those cultural parameters, the individual still has a wide variety of options.

Parkyn (1976) has argued that there are universal criteria for excellence, truth and beauty which transcend cultural limitations. If this is not so, he says 'then there is no point in trying to find individuals who are more gifted than others at recognizing excellence'. He gives as an example the 'universal standards' of good and evil pronounced by the world's most gifted ethical leaders, that is the names associated with the five largest religions of the world today. However, some of us would have little difficulty in distinguishing between these various standards, particularly in their practical aspects.

With regard to the problem of assessing giftedness by means of achievement, Parkyn's summary is brilliantly simple. Firstly, gifted children are expected to pass through the normal processes of development at great speed (no allowance to be made for late developers). Secondly, the gifted have the potential to achieve great insights, beyond those already known. Both these aspects of giftedness are measurable to some extent and should become more so as the knowledge of child development increases with time. However, the absolute value of achievement is not always recognizable by its assessors and I would expect it to retain a subjective element for the foreseeable future.

Achievement aspirations of parents come to a head when the child enters school. If the school has streaming or selection, the hurdles to be jumped are clear and precise and scholastic success can be judged through them. Longitudinal studies in both Britain and America have concluded that early signs of mastery and performance motivation in a child are highly effective predictions of future achievement. (Moss and Kagan, 1961; Douglas, 1968.) There are some sex differences, however. Boys appear to be more achievement orientated than girls and show it earlier; mothers rather than fathers seem to promote it.

Terman and Oden (1959) followed up their sample of gifted children to see how well they had achieved. To do this, they divided their gifted adults into the A group – who had fulfilled their earlier promise – and the C group – who had not made use of their intellectual ability. Comparisons were made on the basis of 200 items of information, secured for 150 subects in each group between 1921 and 1941. In adulthood the As were found to be more interested in vocational matters, politics, social life and literature. Family backgrounds were also different; for the As:

Parents and siblings had more formal education.
Graduate fathers were three times as common.
Fathers were twice as often professional.
Their homes had twice as many books.
The educational tradition of the family was much stronger.
They were better adjusted, both socially and personally.
Separation and divorce between parents was half as common.

In a nutshell:

'Factors other than intellect appear to be highly involved in achievement, and among these factors social and personal adjustment seem to be relatively important.'

The home environments which Terman described for his Californian highly achieving gifted children were the same as I found for English highly achieving gifted children (Chapter 4). Although Terman was measuring adult achievement and I was investigating children, the results are so similar that these children seem very likely to attain the same degree of notable achievement in adult life as the Terman children did. In fact, from the point of view of achievement, gifted children seem to be just as affected by home circumstances as normal children.

There are probably two principal reasons why children develop a strong desire for scholastic achievement (Mussen *et al.,* 1969). Firstly, there is a strong wish to please parents, which is particularly effective if the parents encourage the process, or place most value on intellectual interests. However, encouragement can also be negative, such as that which induces guilt feelings, and carried to excess, encouragement can work against the feeling for achievement. Secondly, there is a strong identification with parents. When parents are seen as being of high intellectual stature and are also able to communicate with the child, identification can be relatively easy, though punitive parents discourage identification. However, children who identify strongly with their parents when there is no basis in reality are over-identifying and must inevitably suffer disappointment.

Studies of achievement are almost always concerned with academic results; other areas, such as social or physical achievement, are little documented. Perhaps it is because the researchers concerned have all been academic. Because of the implicit values in academic achievement, it can be seen to be related to social class values; children from professional or otherwise successful middle-class families achieve significantly better than children from poorly placed families. The traditional middle-class values of education, work improvement and individual success, along with a willingness to move house, are all conducive to higher achievement in the child. The relationship between social class and achievement orientation is in fact well documented in Britain.

## Assessment in practice

Before specific assessment begins, it is essential to be aware of the aims and objectives to which a child's learning is supposed to be directed. Part of an objective measuring procedure is to know how far along this line the child has progressed. There are many teachers and parents who find it difficult, if not 'cold-blooded', to define objectives before they start to teach. They feel that this definition will make education into an impersonal form of training and remove the delicate human relationship between adult and child. Many educational aims are considered to be intangible and therefore both unstatable and un-measurable. Such aims would be, for example, attitudes or values which might not appear till later in life. These intangible long-term outcomes of teaching certainly exist, but they are not all that is taught to a child. Teaching also involves instruction, that is the passing on of information which has to be seen by others to have been received.

Skills are involved in learning and it is a part of assessment to measure these skills in relation to the students, as well as the material to be covered. If parrot-like repetition of information is all that is aimed for in assessment, the task is relatively easy. But assessment of the ability to apply critical thinking skills requires more cunning measurement. Critical thinking can only be defined as an aspect of a subject matter. Without this understanding of the whole area under consideration, we cannot know what has taken place during the teaching. The aims of the course and the skills needed to get there are part of the same learning and of the same assessment.

The techniques which we used in assessment will affect the resulting measurement. Continuing the same example as before, if the repetition of information only is measured by a simple yes/no answer to questions, then the critical thinking skills will be missed, but if questions are included which involve critical discussion of the subject matter, it will enable an assessment to be made of those skills. The result of a yes/no and essay-type assessment can be quite different.

It is possible that different types of the assessment may have to be given more importance than others in order to 'balance' the picture. For example, if a school has been engaged in a particular course of teaching, but an epidemic of measles causes it to be closed temporarily, then the assessment of the pupil's learning would have to recognize the absence of teaching in that time. The marks due to the missing part of the course could be statistically 'weighted' or inflated to the size they would presumably have been, had there not been an outbreak of measles.

Large-scale assessment, such as that made by a local education authority or a national survey, has its own particular problems. In particular, the two basic assumptions on which it is based are arguable. Firstly, that developmental norms which are obtained for any age-group are valid measures to which an individual may be compared and that deviation from that norm is an indication of problems to come. Secondly, that with an active and suitable education the potential problems can be prevented or at least ameliorated.

It is often argued, particularly with regard to gifted children, that if they do not receive special education, they will not satisfy their potential and become frustrated. This progresses naturally from the first assumption – that deviance from the measured ability norm is potentially unhealthy. The second assumption – that exceptional children need exceptional education in order to cope with life – follows from the first. Both of these assumptions involve a concept of almost superhuman responsibility on the part of the adult for the child's welfare. It also implies a belief that what is average is synonymous with contentment. But of course, average ability in any direction does not necessarily mean a lack of problems.

Gifted children are often said to demand, by their very existence, a heavier burden of responsibility from their guardians than normal children. This is said to be because their potential for learning is greater, but their potential for learning the 'wrong' things is also greater; their potential power is greater, and hence their potential misuse of power. Assessment is always used as the basis of intervention in order to change a child's education or life pattern. It is always made with reference to a norm and action is taken on the discovery of deviance from a norm. A gifted child must, by definition, be deviant; intervention must be affected by social attitudes to that particular deviance.

## Assessment in schools

Effort and achievement in school are not of course restricted to the pupils, since teaching is as vital a part of school activities as learning. But to assess teaching is to question its effect within the context of the school's avowed aims. Assessment in schools cannot be understood without evaluation of what is taught, i.e. the curriculum. The 'open' curriculum is what is recognized and stated as being taught, such as geography or history, but equally important is the 'hidden' curriculum which is not always recognized. This includes such old standbys as patriotism, moral duty and physical bearing, as well as the 'affective' values such as imaginativeness and creativity. The hidden curriculum is extremely difficult to assess, although it is of considerable importance in the formation of children's social and psychological perceptions.

## Teacher achievement

Research into teacher achievement in Britain is particularly difficult, because of the traditional privacy of the classroom. Nevertheless enquiry does take place into the effectiveness of teaching, which occasionally results in changes of teaching method. Some of the traditional didactic means by which teachers convey their messages to pupils have certainly been found wanting.

The talking activity of explanation, which forms the main part of a teacher's day, has been found to be a relatively inefficient teaching method (Morrison and McIntyre, 1969). Vital facts or essential principles are often missing in explanatory lessons. Only the more gifted children can cope with a jigsaw lacking some of its parts; many other children fail to grasp the thread of an argument.

Teachers give varying amounts of attention to different pupils in a class, quite unrelated to the requirements of teaching or learning. The sensitivity of approach needed to respond to individual requirements and cries for help calls for a higher level of perceptual skills than many teachers possess. Attention from the teacher may be misunderstood by particular pupils in a way which is detrimental to their self-concepts, and to the view held of them by the rest of the class. A gifted child who shoots his hand up to answer most of the questions put to the class might be told not to put his hand up again that lesson, because the teacher may perceive him as occupying too much of her attention. This 'rejection' of the child can only serve to alienate him from classroom activities and from his classmates.

In ethological terms, the teacher is – by the nature of his job – in a dominant position. Non-verbal signs and signals which he gives are interpreted by the pupils in terms of his leadership position. For any pupil the posture, proximity, facial expression, tone of voice, etc. of the teacher are all important. Behind his desk or 'boundary', the teacher is safe in his own territory, but good eye contact from him indicates warmth and friendliness.

Different and distinguishable atmospheres are present in different schools. They stem largely from the attitudes held within the school hierarchy. Satisfied teachers are kinder to pupils and teach better, while pupils' perceptions are affected by the attitudes of their teachers. In this way, gifted children are sometimes seen by teachers as unwelcome, if not threatening. Picking up such feelings, their schoolmates would then react accordingly and the child suffer from lack of friends, and from being 'different'.

A good teacher is able and willing to incorporate at least some of the findings and practical implications of educational psychological research into his teaching. Attitude formation is a particularly important by-product of teaching any subject, while self-awareness and knowledge of what one is doing are indispensible aspects of teaching in general. But there are more teachers who, because of their own personality problems or immaturity, are unable to bring this about in the classroom.

## Pupil achievement

In whatever manner the performance of pupils is assessed at school, whether by marks or words, it acts as a form of feedback. Pupils understand how well they are succeeding on the school programme, teachers see how effective their teaching has been, parents make their judgements on the results and employers eventually have something to go by. The assessment of performance is also of concern to central and local government, being used in the development of educational policy and the allocation of resources.

Most assessment of pupils is initiated and practised by the school staff. This 'internal' assessment is not co-ordinated nationally or even within the same local education authority in Britain. But there is an effective system of inspection for every school, which is nationally organized through Her Majesty's Inspectors (HMIs).

Many of the tests which can be used by teachers, though not designed by them, were standardized years ago and the standards of performance on which they were based have changed. These tests are also subject to educational 'fashion'; they were, on the whole, designed to reflect the curriculum of their day and are no longer appropriate to current classroom practice and emphasis.

The British Government has recently formed an Assessment of Performance Unit (APU) which is attempting to make available a *national* picture of some aspects of school performance. Though it will not produce reports on individual children, it should go a long way towards enabling individual children to be assessed in terms of national norms. This should make the identification of achievement in gifted children easier.

There is a growing feeling for 'accountability' in education, which involves increased assessment of what pupils have learned within different types of education. It is possibly the natural result of the recognition that resources are limited and that they should be employed to their greatest efficiency. It is impossible to imagine that there will be a time when the regular individual testing by teachers of their pupils is replaced by nationally ordained tests. This day-to-day assessment is part and parcel of good teaching and should involve all aspects of a child's work and behaviour. Assessment of this nature is not only a measure of performance, but is a means of giving practical experience in the application of the skills which have been taught.

The Warnock Report (DES, 1978a) has pointed out that some children may escape the assessment procedures normally used by teachers. Weaknesses or incipient problems are not always accurately identifiable by the teacher – neither for that matter is giftedness when it is not specifically allied with achievement. This report recommended that a form of screening organized by the local education authority could go a long way towards picking up exceptional children who may be heading for problems in school. But there is always the danger of over-testing children, a danger of which some American educationalists are already complaining. This includes exhausting the children's enthusiam for learning and distorting the curriculum to fit the tests, thereby lowering rather than raising standards.

Objective achievement testing in schools is relatively easy, since the accumulation of information is readily available to this process. But reasoning or transfer – less objective aspects of achievement – are not as amenable to rating. Achievement can only be measured in respect of the goals of specific teaching and the expectations of the teacher as to how well the child is expected to do. Success and failure in respect of achievement are always relative terms.

There are benefits to pupils from achievement tests as short-term goals, as learning experiences in themselves and as a form of feedback. In psychological terms, where children receive encouraging feedback it should act as reinforcement to their learning habits and they should then go on to achieve more and more. However, if the reinforcement is negative and the child feels herself to be a failure, she may give up the struggle or just keep a low profile till she can leave school. Logically, highly achieving gifted children can only be more successful at every test, while poorly achieving gifted children or less capable children will in time desert the academic system. This does in fact seem to happen and in this way the achievement test acts to increase the divisions in children's attainments.

The achievement test is often used as a segregator without reference to the rest of the child, as in selection for some highly academic schools, for example. The gifted child from a poor background or poor primary education is thus debarred from mixing with his peers. Often, the results of these tests are used by a school as the sole indications to parents of the child's progress. The parent is not always able to interpret the same meanings, from an isolated mark, that the school intended. Thus, the tests may give a false picture of school achievement. Even apparently objective marking can be affected by a teacher's dislike of a pupil, or by a wish to put him down.

Continuous assessment is becoming more popular, but also has its limitations. The teacher keeps a record over the year of the quality of a pupil's essays, assignments and general educational progression. But it is not as clear-cut as a test and has all the built-in biases of being marked by one person, who also has a form of emotional relationship with the pupil.

Self-evaluation is perhaps the least used aspect of education, yet it is an important one, particularly for gifted children. All pupils who are partners in their own learning – helping to set up objectives, devising routes by which to reach them, etc. – will obtain the greatest benefit from self-evaluation, which is their very own feedback. It also provides the pupil with an important lesson in understanding his own learning processes and understanding himself – a vital part of education. But the validity of self-evaluation is uncertain, since some people inevitably tend to over- or under-estimate themselves. Pupils will need expert help all the way, in both insight and self-confidence.

## Research methods

Every kind of investigation stands or falls on the quality of three essential procedures. These are, firstly, the choice of subjects to be investigated, secondly, the design of the enquiry and, thirdly, the interpretation of its results. The nature of all three procedures can be related to the reasons the research was carried out, although these may not always be the stated reasons. If any of either the research procedures or the underlying reasons for their choice are doubtful, then so are the reported results.

There are also two well known grounds on which an investigation may be judged. These should be critically applied to all aspects of any piece of research.

(1)   Validity - does the investigation measure what it is supposed to measure?

(2)   Reliability - can it give the same results in the same circumstances every time?

## Problems of selection

In selecting a group of children on the basis of their level of ability, it is impossible to record every aspect of a child's performance. In that case, it is necessary to take a sample of this performance; a situation has to be arranged where the child's ability or level of achievement has an opportunity to show itself. While such a sample allows an estimate to be made of the child's.overall ability, the accuracy of the estimate depends on the adequacy of the sample.

With the progress of time, new researchers become aware of the mistakes of older ones; their faults may simply have been due to lack of knowledge which we now have, so that the earlier work seems limited in scope. But these limitations were enhanced by the fashionable concerns of the time. An example is the work of Terman and his associates (1925) on gifted children in California; his sampling method would not be acceptable today, as his research population was virtually all white and middle-class. He began this work at a time of intense concern.with the nature of intelligence, but without our present-day recognition of the effects on intelligence tests scores of different social settings. However, he worked within the ethos of his time, just as we must work within ours.

Many studies in the past, directed by university teachers, have used students as samples and generalized from them to the rest of the population. It is still done, for reasons of economy and convenience, but the results will always be doubtful when they are used in relation to anyone but university students.

A considerable problem in the selection of children as gifted, for purposes of study, is the means by which they are to be selected. There is always argument as to what to look for as the distinguishing features of gifted children (outlined in Chapter 1). Furthermore, there are even doubts about who should select them. The National Children's Bureau (Hitchfield, 1973) used no less than three questionable methods, given below, in their nationwide survey of Britain:

(1) The results of the Goodenough Draw-a-man test (Goodenough, 1926). This test is recognized as being particularly affected by social and cultural differences.

(2) School attainment and teacher's recommendation. Fortunately, teachers are human beings, but because of their humanity they are not reliable sources of pupil assessment. It is well recognized from other studies that teacher assessment is influenced by, for example, the child's appearance, or the status of her parents (Freeman, 1975; Morrison and McIntyre, 1972). Gifted children who do not conform to teacher expectations and are not achieving well at school can be missed by teachers. In a study by Pegnato and Birch (1966) in a junior high school in Pittsburgh, USA, only 41 of the 91 children with 'Stanford–Binet' IQs of 136 or more were nominated by their teachers as gifted.

> 'Not only were more than half of the gifted missed, but a breakdown of these children referred to as gifted by the teachers were not in the gifted or superior range, but in the average intelligence range on the Binet.' (p. 78)

In addition, they found that more than 10% of the gifted children in their study were achieving less well in school than they could.

(3) Parent identification. The Bureau wrote to papers and magazines, asking parents to nominate their gifted children. This voluntary sub-sample was mixed with the other two selected sub-samples, without quibble. The validity of this last section is very doubtful as it depends on the readership of the different types of journals used and on the willingness and capability of the respondent adults to put pen to paper.

An interesting study was carried out on gifted children in Southport, England (Tempest, 1974). Seven-year old children were first selected by a group intelligence test (Young, 1966), and then by the Wechsler Intelligence Scale for Children (Wechsler, 1949) along with several other tests. Although well aware of the problems of selecting children as gifted, Tempest excluded from his sample all children attending private schools. This must have been a notable omission from his population of children in an affluent town, which has many private schools. As my own research (p. 205) has shown that gifted children in affluent areas are more likely to attend private schools, the Southport sample may not be typical of gifted children, even in Southport. The selected children there were given special education for four years for their particular abilities, by a non-specialist teacher. During this time, there was virtually no contact between the researchers and the children's homes; the study also lacked any adequately matched control group. There has, however, been a follow-up investigation and the results of this may well be of interest.

Selecting children for a special programme for mathematically precocious children, the team at Johns Hopkins University (Stanley, Keating and Fox, 1974) used a competition as their basis of selection. They rejected teacher or parent referral as 'insufficient' and did not screen the children before the competition. The element of competition is very much a part of the North American culture and would probably select those children who are not only mathematically precocious, but also keen to succeed. As a consequence, the project would be more likely to be successful since potential drop-outs would either have refused to enter the competition or have made less effort at winning it.

The Russians have a system of selection for their schools for talented youth which seems to make use of every available method (Dunstan, 1977), constituting a form of talent-scouting. The Central Music School in Moscow, for instance, draws its pupils nationwide, though clearly an attempt to pick out the musical best from four million seven-year olds is an impossibility. It recruits through the national and local media, a process which requires parents to put their children forward. But it also has provision for musically gifted children who are orphaned or in special homes. About 200 children will come to the school for tests and of these 30 will be selected. Whether because of this wide method of selection, or from what happens afterwards, the children in the specialist schools achieve spectacularly well.

# Problems of design

It is of essential importance, when an investigation is being planned, for the researcher to decide what it is he wants to measure. For example, in developing a procedure to look at the progress of gifted children in school, it is necessary to be sure of what is wanted from the exercise – measurement of ability or achievement. A school achievement test may only measure the effectiveness of the teaching method; it may show that pupils have plenty of information, but lack the ability to apply it. On the other hand, the procedure may be sufficiently cunning to reach under the teaching and actually define the children's natural abilities. The results of any investigation, therefore, are dependent on its design. As an example of contentious design, Professor Bennett sent questionnaires to 800 junior schools in the North West of England (Bennett, 1976). On the basis of their responses, he divided the schools into two groups of teaching styles – primarily formal or primarily informal. Responses to questionnaires, though, are not necessarily the same as the reality these describe; what one professes is not always the same as what one can be observed to practise. Then, in order to measure the progress of the children in these schools, he tested their academic achievement with paper and pencil tests of school subjects. Not surprisingly, perhaps, the pupils with the least formal type of teaching did the least well on these 'formal' tests. He did not report the social background of the children in the final selection of schools. As schools tend to draw on their surrounding social areas, this is a matter of great importance to the success of different teaching styles – higher social class parents tend to prefer more formal teaching styles. It was concluded that formal teaching was, on the whole, a better bet than informal teaching, but because of the contentiousness of the design, the conclusion is not entirely acceptable to other educational researchers. However, it seems to have brought political joy to the hearts of many.

Doubt about method does not always produce doubt about conclusions, though. Piaget's investigations were basically conversations and observations of his own and other middle-class Swiss children, but his conclusions have spread into the educational theory and practice of most of the world.

Another theory which has influenced the thinking of at least the Western World, and which is based on shaky methodology, is that of Basil Bernstein in London (Bernstein, 1960). His hypothesis of the language differential between classes has promoted a huge edifice of theory and research. It is particularly important in the selection of gifted children, as the verbal bias of intelligence scales towards the middle classes is now almost universally accepted and must affect just who is considered to be gifted. Briefly, Bernstein claims that working class children are brought up to speak in a limited 'public code', while the middle classes (which include teachers), use an elaborate 'formal code'. As they progress through the educational system, working class children are described as becoming more and more conceptually distant from the world of their educators, slipping further down the educational slope. By this logic, there must be many more gifted middle than working class children.

Bernstein's original study in 1960 compared verbal ability in boys from the most exclusive private schools with that in working boys given some time off by their employers to attend a day-release course. He found the boys who were still attending full-time education in their exclusive schools to be very much more articulate than the day-release boys. This was not a surprising result from such a comparison, but the colossal weight of theory which followed, about the differences between the social classes, was based only on this research. Further work has since been done by Bernstein and others, with varying results.

## Problems of interpretation

An interpretation is, in effect, the researcher's response to findings. When the subjects of the research have made their reactions to questions, it is the person responsible for the investigation who must then give the final return. The interpretation is always subjective; it cannot be otherwise. A computer can only decipher information by means of the statistical programme which it is given; it cannot respond sympathetically nor work on hunches. The human being is always the final interpreter, who will go on to make the decisions for the next operation. Gunnar Myrdal, the philosopher, summarized this situation (Myrdal, 1970):

'Facts do not organize themselves into concepts and theories just by being looked at. Questions must be asked before answers are given. The questions are all expressions of our interest in the world; they are at bottom evaluations. There is an inescapable a priori element in all scientific work.'

Some types of research are much more open to subjective interpretation than others. The interview, for example, even when the questions are rigorously pre-tested and fixed in position beforehand, is open to the effects of personal interaction between the people involved.

The objective style of testing is very popular in America at present, due to the large amount of testing which is carried out and the ease of marking this kind of test. Essentially, it has right answers to the questions and the child has to show that he knows these. The answers must be predictable for the test to be objective. Essay-type tests allow a freedom of response and oblige the child to organize the information, as well as express it. However an essay-type test or creative endeavour by a child can be assessed by different judges as anything from terrible to brilliant. There are ways round these entirely subjective interpretations, such as taking the average opinion of a panel of judges or by mixing objective and subjective tests.

A particularly controversial interpretation of his own research was presented by Jensen (1972). He had compared the intelligence levels of different races, a prickly enough activity in itself. His evidence was interpreted as demonstrating social class and racial differences in intelligence test results. Although, clearly, scientific argument must be restricted to that which is measurable, no instruments have yet been devised which, even added together, can encompass all psychological function. For instance, there is the consistent and well documented over-representation of first-born and only children among high achievers and the gifted. Jensen dismisses this unexplained phenomenon as being 'probably biological'. But what about parental expectation and why do twins have a lower IQ than single children?

Jensen matched black and white children for socio-economic level and measured their IQs. He found that the black children's IQs covered the whole range, but that their average IQ was about 15 points lower than that of the matched white children. He interpreted this as meaning that black intelligence was different from white intelligence and so could not be measured on the same tests. He proposed that different forms of education, more appropriate to their kind of intelligence, should be given to black children. There should be less conceptual flights of fancy and more rote learning for them.

This raises many questions, particularly of the middle-class subjects. We must assume that since the abolition of slavery, these black people have made great upward progress, whereas the white subjects may or may not have moved their social position. If the black population are bearing the double handicaps of 15 points less IQ and probably racial prejudice, they have done remarkably well.

*101*

Conversely, if black and white middle-class people of the same IQ were compared, it could be interpreted that the whites were under-achieving. If a comparison were to be made between American black people in their predominantly white society and an all-black stratified society such as Ghana or the French West Indies, the results might prove to be interesting.

The practical proposals resulting from Jensen's interpretation of the material are quite unacceptable. Selecting educational methods and standards by skin colour cannot ever be justified. Teaching children as individuals does not involve a statistical knowledge of their dubious genetic potential.

The implications of the interpretation of Bennett's work, mentioned above (p. 99), that formal education is better than informal, can be serious for educational policy. Most unfortunately, his is almost the only research to have been carried out into styles of teaching. Consequently, the conclusion that there should be a return to more formality in teaching holds the stage in Britain at present. It is only a human faith in the newer, more open and supposedly more creative type of teaching that fuels its continued growth. There is certainly a crying need here for further research. If teaching is truly open and informal, each child learning at her own pace, there would theoretically be no question at all of separate education for the gifted.

## Problems of confirmation

It is always a deficiency in research on child development that follow-up and replication studies are few. The one-shot research is unfortunately typical, but a longer term view is necessary in order to assess the validity and reliability of the original results. Rewriting the same information in a variety of ways is not the same thing. Unfortunately, though, our academic system in the Western World is not geared to long-term research; most investigation is done by postgraduate students in search of higher degrees or researchers on short-term contracts. Tenured academic staff have their teaching duties and are limited in the funds which they can get to employ help for their research projects. At the moment, the funding available for studies of gifted children is low.

Because of the way research has to be carried out, there is a plethora of small samples, thereby increasing the possibility of error and biased results. These small, atypical studies bear little relationship to one another and are necessarily limited in scope. Group classifications of children in terms of the mass of material produced often appear to be arbitrary. This results in a serious loss of information which could have been obtained, had there been communication and organization between individuals before their studies were begun. There is also a tendency to generalize from these small studies beyond their immediate subjects simply because there are so few large-scale studies to which they may be referenced. Sometimes the selected gifted children are studied without controls of non-gifted children at all and very often important factors such as home background, test conditions or sex are not recognized as effective variables. In the organization of a research project in child development, convenience and availability to the researcher are unlikely to be the most accurate reflection of the life circumstances of the children concerned.

Almost all research work, both with children and adults, has been restricted to men. But even so, there are indications that creativity and thought processes between boys and girls may function differently. Differences have been found with respect to female creativity and the social desirability of what girls made and did. Responses in creativity of boys and girls have also been found to vary with the sex of the experimenter.

In order to give a full picture of the gifted child, studies which are both broadly based and longitudinal are vital. The questions of burnt-out potential or problems of early precocity, for example, can only be answered in that way. Developmental variables and the interaction of personality, cognitive and environmental effects are long-term processes. Knowledge of them in gifted children is essential to any theory of giftedness and though there is some developmental evidence, it is not yet enough or systematized. Almost all studies rely on particular intellectual traits, with little regard for personality styles and the world the children live in.

## INTELLIGENCE

As psychological understanding of children increases, the concept of intelligence is being viewed afresh. The older, narrower definitions of it are giving way to the idea of a relatively more flexible system of intellectual development. Since one member, the IQ, is no longer being regarded as sufficiently descriptive of the richness and variety of mental ability, tests now being devised are based instead on the concept of a 'profile', notably the yet to be published British Intelligence Scales

(Elliott, 1974). However parents and teachers continue to use the numbers to identify children, often with some innocence as to even which test was used. Tests of verbal ability have been seen by myself to be used in schools as if they were intelligence tests; group tests used in schools often give a lower score than individual tests given by psychologists. Intelligence tests seem to measure conventional scholastic ability well enough, but doubt has been raised as to whether they can measure unusual ability. If an intelligence test is flexible, without rigidly standardized answers to questions, it should be able to measure unusual ability. But then what is the value of measuring say a musically talented child on an intelligence test?

Intelligence itself is a form of behaviour and as such is capable of being developed. Some aspects of intelligence, such as reasoning or learning ability, are known to develop continuously from birth, if not before. Suitable experience is necessary for this development; without it, some facets of intelligence might never develop and even atrophy. Not all the rich potential of a baby's inherent intelligence can be developed though, since life circumstances vary for every individual.

## Some measures

The most widely used intelligence test is the contemporary version of the one designed by Alfred Binet in Paris at the beginning of the century, which successfully predicted the scholastic performances of French schoolchildren. Reissued by Terman at Stanford University in California, it again proved to be a reliable predictor, this time of the performances of American school children. It was revised again in 1961 and is now known as the Terman–Merril revision of the Stanford–Binet Intelligence Test. It is currently being re-standardized on British schoolchildren.

The test is based on the growth of children's knowledge with age. They are asked questions of increasing difficulty, until they can no longer give the correct answers. The level that each child reaches on the test is known as her mental age, which is the age at which most children reach that level of answering correctly. The child's mental age is divided by her real, chronological age to provide her intelligence quotient, or IQ. (A quotient is the result of arithmetical division). Because the test measures a high proportion of learned ability it is a first class measure of academic ability, but does not necessarily provide a true picture of general mental ability.

The Stanford–Binet is so widely used that other tests are often tried out on it, to see how well they can predict in comparison to this well established measure. Thus, very many current tests of IQ bear an uncanny resemblance to the original Stanford–Binet, so that whatever these intelligence tests measure, it is likely to be the same. During its various redesignings, any item which appeared to discriminate between the sexes was replaced by one on which boys and girls scored equally. It is the only readily available and well recognized test which can identify children in the very high ranges of ability. Measured intelligence on this test ranges up to IQ 170. The Wechsler intelligence scales are the next best known, internationally trusted tests. These scales were devised by David Wechsler during 1939–49 and there are several of them, designed for different age-groups. They were not built up item by item like the Stanford–Binet, offering only a single result, but each scale is a 'whole' test in itself. They do, however, correlate highly with the Stanford–Binet results.

Weschler's scales are designed to measure the growth and decline of intellectual ability according to age. The scales are composed of sub-scales of items, involving different tasks to measure different abilities, whatever the mental or chronological age of the child. These separate sub-scores provide flexibility in measurement. He also attempted to eliminate items which seemed to be biased towards either sex, but the sub-tests of the scales do in fact differentiate between the sexes. Boys and girls typically differ in the tasks in which their best scores are obtained.

A version of the Stanford–Binet test has been the basic measure of intelligence in all studies of gifted children since Terman's work in 1925. Its main technical drawback is that the sub-test scores, which make up the final single score, are in different combinations for different mental ages. Because of this, it is not possible to make precise comparisons of specific traits with this test, other than on the vocabulary scale. It is the preciseness of the Wechsler scales and the ease with which verbal and performance scores can be compared that has made this test popular among psychologists. This has been particularly so when the children to be tested have specific problems. In her studies of Young Fluent Readers, Margaret Clark appears to have come across the same problem of choice between the two major intelligence tests as I did myself. She explains that (Clark, 1976):

'Although at first sight it appears that use of the Wechsler Tests provides a comprehensive scale for analysis of intellectual functioning from pre-school to adulthood, there is a weak link around six to seven years of age, which in Britain is often a crucial age for assessment. This weakness became evident when testing the brighter children in this study. While they were still within the range for the norms of the WPPSI (Wechsler) they were in actual fact reaching the ceiling on a number of sub-tests. Several children could have obtained the same final scaled scores or even the same IQ with a much lower level of functioning. For this reason it was decided to retest on the Stanford–Binet Intelligence Scale.'

In fact, Clark tested the fluent readers on both scales and her results are seen below. Where the Wechsler test maximum score was IQ 140, some children were able to score up to IQ 170 on the Stanford–Binet. This latter thus appears to discriminate between children at the higher levels of ability, i.e. to continue where the Wechsler leaves off.

**Comparison of intelligence scores as measured on WPPSI and Stanford–Binet intelligence scales (Clark, 1976, p. 23)**

| Stanford–Binet Freq. at each IQ level | WPPSI Frequencies at each IQ level | | | | | | |
|---|---|---|---|---|---|---|---|
| | 90+ | 100+ | 110+ | 120+ | 130+ | 140+ | Totals |
| 170+ | — | — | — | — | 2 | 1 | 3 |
| 160+ | — | — | — | — | 1 | 1 | 2 |
| 150+ | — | — | 1 | 2 | 1 | — | 4 |
| 140+ | — | — | 6 | 2 | 4 | — | 12 |
| 130+ | — | 3 | 1 | 1 | — | — | 5 |
| 120+ | 1 | 1 | 1 | — | 1 | — | 4 |
| 110+ | — | — | 1 | 1 | — | — | 2 |
| 100+ | — | — | — | — | — | — | — |
| Totals | 1 | 4 | 10 | 6 | 9 | 2 | 32 |

There is sometimes the complaint that the individual one-to-one testing which is obligatory with the Stanford–Binet will allow a child to be brighter than he or she would be in a group test. This may well be so, but in the circumstances of my own study, all the children were tested individually and so there could be no test-circumstance differences between the target and control groups. I could only agree with Clark (1978) that:

'the skill of the tester was required only in maintaining and matching the child's high level of functioning rather than stimulating it'.

The Stanford–Binet does have a heavy verbal emphasis, especially at the upper levels (Vernon, 1961). This can be seen simply by looking over the test. It has also been seen as a test of 'intellectual attainment with a high verbal content' (Phillips and Bannon, 1968). Some pre-school intervention studies in America have even used the test as both a baseline test and a measure of the effectiveness of the teaching programme. But the Wechsler scales are equally over-emphatic on mathematical ability at the upper levels, as Hitchfield (1973, Appendix) discovered. The choice then, especially in testing gifted children, is between the lesser of two biases. Other available intelligence tests are not dissimilar in make-up, but are less well known and standardized than these two. The only alternative is not to test at all, which would leave the reader rather short on information.

The main reasons for choosing the Stanford–Binet in preference to the Wechsler Intelligence Scale for Children in a study of gifted children can be summarised as follows:

(i)     The Stanford–Binet measures children more precisely in the higher ranges of ability than the Wechsler. It ranges up to 170 IQ, whereas the Wechsler overall IQ only reaches 140. Measurement of the top intellectual range is clearly important and Wechsler himself doubts the efficiency of his scales at the higher levels (Wechsler, 1949).

(ii)    The Stanford-Binet is much less likely than the Wechsler to discriminate between the sexes on grounds of general ability.

(iii)   It is the most widely used test of intelligence, with the longest history. Consequently, it has more accumulated evidence and interpretive data than other tests. Behaviour which can be expected from a Stanford–Binet IQ score is well founded on experience.

The Raven's Progressive Matrices is a British test which has been designed to cover the 'whole range of intellectual development from infancy to maturation' (Raven, 1965). It is non-verbal and 'probably the most culture-free test of general intelligence yet devised by psychologists' (Jensen, 1973a). It effectively measures a high element of general intelligence and is affected very little by the socio-economic status of the subjects.

This test is designed to measure the ability to grasp relationships. Unlike many other tests of ability, it does not include the recall of specific learned information, such as vocabulary or general knowledge. The intention is to measure productive, rather than reproductive, thinking and because scholastic attainment as such is relatively unimportant in this test, illiterate and unschooled people can score highly on it.

In the Raven's Matrices, the subject has to replace the missing part of a matrix or pattern from a numbered choice of pattern pieces; there is no penalty for guessing. The basic idea is very simple and the earliest problems in the series can be solved by children under five years old. The test comes in three forms – a coloured version for young children, a standard version and an advanced version, suitable for university graduates. Using this test over a wide age and ability range, it is possible to obtain a uniformity of measurement which can be used as a basis for comparison of such subjects.

The Raven's Matrices is widely used as a group test, although it can be given in a one-to-one situation. It is untimed, so that speed of working (a dubious factor of other ability scales) is irrelevant. Intellectual capacity is not confused with intellectual efficiency.

An additional bonus is that children find the test enjoyable. As there was such a large battery of tests in the research project described ahead (Chapter 4), there was always the danger of boredom and of less than full co-operation. The Raven's test had been standardized on British children and so the percentile figures given could be considered as the most reliable ones available for this sample of children.

## Arguments about measuring intelligence

There is always some sort of moral stance made when one human being measures another; the standards being used for measurement and the reasons for doing it become open to dispute. Though IQ tests have been around for some time, considerable controversy surrounds their use and interpretation.

# Heredity and environment

The longest standing argument against measuring intelligence is that IQ tests are culturally discriminating. In America, they are widely used to 'track' and sort pupils into different types of education within the school; 85% of high schools 'track' students into courses with different curricula and most elementary schools are the same. This is becoming less common in Britain as segregated education in general has become less acceptable. But in America, the trend is probably now towards some form of segregated education for all children, in terms of intelligence.

It is contended in America that black children especially suffer most from this 'tracking', as they are too often mistakenly placed in 'educationally mentally retarded' (EMR) classes on the basis of low IQ scores. For example, in 1977 blacks were 66% of the EMR students in San Francisco, but only 27.5% of the total school population; the figures for other states are not dissimilar. Blacks are fighting the use of IQ tests in the courts, claiming that they are a form of insidious and effective discrimination which is being used against them.

The question of race and its relationship to intelligence (as presently measured) is the most sensitive issue in modern educational theory. The most notable and contentious figure in this field is Jensen (1973a), whose research results gave evidence that blacks on average score 15 points below whites on IQ tests. Is this an accurate reflection of a genetic fact of life, or is it the result of biased testing instruments? Several wide surveys agreeing with Jensen have been published, such as Jencks (1973), Herrnstein (1973) and Eysenck (1973). But criticism of their work has been considerable at many levels. In their wide ranging review of all the research that has been done on the relationship between parents' and children's intelligence, McAskie and Clarke (1976) concluded that:

> 'if any of these reviewers' assessments prove correct (which they might), it will certainly not be due to the care with which they have handled the evidence. Even Jencks' most sophisticated attempt failed to match an elaborate mathematical analysis with a commensurate attention to the nature of the data'.

They also found (McAskie and Clarke, 1976):

> 'that much of the difference among offspring scores is not directly attributable to parental IQ and that some is due to other between-family variables'.

In other words, little real evidence for the genetic transmission of IQ has been found in the work carried out to date. Using sophisticated statistical techniques to 'pull together' the findings of many studies, they concluded that 70–75% of the offspring variance is not *directly* related to IQ. Even when allowance has been made for variance *indirectly* related to parent IQ, 35–45% was still unexplained. They also found that there was no systematic tendency for children of one sex to 'identify' intellectually with a parent of the same or opposite sex. Nor was there a higher relationship between mothers' and children's IQs, on the assumption that mothers spend more time with their children than fathers.

In brief, McAskie and Clarke found that all the available evidence about hereditary or environmental influences on intelligence were statistically unsound. This means that whatever the actual situation is – whether IQ is of primarily genetic origin or is environmentally determined – we cannot say with any confidence that we have reliable evidence for either case.

In his controversial book *The Science and Politics of IQ*, Leon Kamin (1974) describes how intelligence tests have been used in good faith as tools of discrimination against unacceptable races and the poor. He exposes inconsistencies and improbabilities in research evidence which uses intelligence tests. IQ, he says, is the end-product of some man's social views 'dressed in the trappings of science rather than politics'. He quotes a report of the United States Public Health service in 1912 to the Ellis Island organization which tested incoming immigrants. 'The test results established that 83% of the Jews, 80% of the Hungarians, 79% of the Italians and 87% of the Russians were "feeble minded".'

This type of evidence is dramatic, but 60 years out of date. Science has progressed considerably since that time, and psychologists today are highly aware of social influences on their work. But we are all too human; in future retrospect, we may be seen to have fallen victim to the social mores of our own times. In fact, IQ tests can never be entirely objective. They are a product of the people who make them – who are themselves members of their own society.

## The make-up of the tests

The thread of all concern about intelligence tests is that they are not measuring intelligence at all, but rather a variety of other aspects of life. Patently, a test is an inventory of behaviour and scores on that basis do predict school achievement very well. But other indices of school achievement could equally well be formed from such environmental factors as fathers' income or the quality of the home and they might well predict equally well; though this has not been tried yet.

The Stanford–Binet test is undoubtedly cumbersome to give and tiresome to take. A young gifted child can consume up to two hours' testing time on this test alone. Certain, less than determined children falter on the way and though a break will suffice to recharge some, others refuse to return to the testing. It is probable that a very positive attitude towards school-like activities and a desire to do well would keep a child going and enhance test performance. In reverse, the child who does not like school or the tester could be at a disadvantage, but this condition could apply to any test. In my research (Chapter 4), this problem was recognized and mitigated by testing the children in the familiarity of their own homes.

The Stanford–Binet test, especially its vocabulary section, is in considerable need of updating. Very few children in my sample for example, knew the word 'brunette' which is only the 14th of 45 words, increasing in difficulty. To do well on a vocabulary test implies an excellent knowledge of English. What is more, the English measured is of a literary rather than a spoken style; the words do not appear in many newspapers or comics, but rather in formal literature. Immigrants or children of poor cultural background will do less well on the verbal aspect of any test which is described as measuring intelligence.

Some items on the Stanford–Binet test measure current social values quite explicitly. As an example, pictures of a woman are shown; one is neat and the other very untidy. The question is: 'Which one is prettier?' and the answer is the tidy one. Many of the required answers appear to be aspects of American Protestantism, such as . . .

Question: 'What's the thing to do if another boy (girl, person) hits you without meaning to do it?'

Wrong answer: 'I would hit them back'.

Throughout, there is a need for the child to find the 'correct' answer; though his behaviour in the playground can be quite different. There are rules to the 'game', which a child may have discovered at leisure in his home, but which others of less socially acceptable homes may have to grasp very quickly in the course of the test. Perhaps this is an unrecognized measure of their intelligence. In fact, the content of these test items makes it fairly sure that it will discriminate among people on the basis of their access to educational opportunities, personal attitudes, and social background rather than intelligence (Cronin *et al.*, 1975).

Similar criticisms apply to the make-up of the Wechsler test. The main difference between the two tests is a heavier emphasis in the Wechsler on performance. But performance can also be seen as testing obedience and motivation; for example, one Wechsler performance sub-scale involves copying marks. The test does not require thinking, but rather motivation, rapport with the tester and obedience. The verbal part of the Wechsler is exactly like that of the Stanford-Binet.

The answers to comprehension questions on the Wechsler also parallel those on the Stanford–Binet. For example . . .
Question: 'Why should a promise be kept?'
Right Answer: 'A promise has the status of an implied contract.'
Wrong Answer: 'You can gain friends by keeping promises.'
It's that game again.

To the extent that it measures intelligence, the Wechsler test appears to be very similar to the Stanford–Binet test. The roots from which most success in life springs, that of class background and social attitudes, are the same ones that provide success in IQ tests. Hence, there is a close relationship between success and IQ score. Several studies have shown that economic success in the United States correlates highly with length of time in education, rather than with how well a person did while he was there. There seems to be little relationship between grades in school and success afterwards. But the success of the high IQ scorers does not of itself make the tests valid measures of intelligence; rather, they are indicators of life opportunities.

None the less, it is only through these tests – the Stanford–Binet in particular – that intellectually gifted children have a chance to be identified in the light of our present knowledge of measurement. The tests do have legitimate values and applications and should be recogniz-ed at least for what they are. Within our present system, they do provide a highly reliable measure of prediction of a child's capacity to benefit from school instruction.

A test can only take a sample of behaviour. During the test, a child gives evidence of how well he has accepted and understood the processes of learning offered to him. Attempts to test experience-free intelligence have not been entirely successful; learning in itself affects the innate ability to learn. Testing of inherited ability would have to take place even before the experience of birth. To say that intelligence, if it is to be measured at all, should be measured separately from environmental influences is to carry the argument about 'fairness' to the point of theoretical and practical absurdity.

One answer to this dilemma is to throw out the tests, along with all the information that has been gathered about them. Then, there would be no means of assessing children's intellectual abilities and chance or random factors would again be foremost in deciding how children should be educated. This was the situation before the advent of intelligence tests. No even remotely objective help was given to children in this respect.

School systems differentiate in myriad ways between pupils, and some of these ways magnify the differences between them. Schools produce different results in different pupils; inevitably the system has its failures as well as its successes. The subtle pressures within an institution like a school reflect the social pressures of the society which supports it.

The IQ measure can and does enable children, who would otherwise be regulated only by social or random pressures, to function at somewhere near their own level. Even as it stands, it can identify children who merit special attention and who would otherwise have sunk without trace in the educational process. Teachers' opinions alone are notoriously unreliable. The IQ test is still the only relatively objective structure which can give support and direction to a child in a sea of opinions. But the value of a test will always depend on the discretion with which it is used.

## Sex differences in intelligence

There has been a lack of consistency in the results of research studies which have compared adults of the two sexes for intelligence. Certainly, it is not possible to conclude that one sex is more intelligent than the other, but there is some evidence, which is not universally accepted, for a greater *range* of intelligence among boys. This would mean that there are relatively both more low ability and more gifted boys than girls, which would fit in with everyday observation that men are greater achievers and that schools for the mentally retarded contain a relative excess of boys. However, there are many and varied socio-cultural reasons for these sex disparities, which undermine the apparent meaning of what can be perceived. We only see the way things are, not how they came to be that way, nor how they might change with different perception. For example, the reason that there are more boys than girls in schools for the mentally retarded may be due to the greater attention paid to boys' development. It is possible, judging from other identified attitudes to children, that a mentally retarded girl is more likely to be kept at home than a similar boy.

Accumulated evidence during this century has shown that there is a reciprocal relationship between education and measured intelligence. When Wechsler first devised his scales in 1939 in the USA, he found slight but positive differences in favour of females at all ages (Wechsler, 1939). However, later revisions showed a superiority of men over women; these changes are explicable in terms of education received.

Before the Second World War, women in the USA in every age-category had completed more years of education than their brothers. But during the forties, the average number of years of education completed by young American males increased by almost two years, to exceed the average education level of women. Later, during the sixties, males continued to exceed women in their age-group in length of education. Both decades show a change in the educational advantages of males, which were accurately reflected in Wechsler's normative data during the time. Other studies at the same time produced the same results, but more recent reports show no sex differences in intelligence (Bayley, 1957).

The reason for this change in educational level between men and women was undoubtedly the concern of the United States Government to reward ex-servicemen by conferring educational advantage; other countries did the same after World War II. This involved financial support and exemptions from service for those attending higher education. Thus, the incentives for males to enter higher education have increased over the years as ex-servicemen continue to be produced (e.g. Korea and Vietnam), but have applied only to a minimal extent to females. It can be seen from these considerable data that subjects who receive the most formal education do best on tests of intelligence (Kipnis, 1976).

Differences in intelligence have been seen clearly and regularly when normal boys and girls are compared at different ages. Feminine superiority in IQ is notable in childhood, but this is followed by changes in levels of specific abilities which bring about male equality of IQ and for some actual male superiority. Probably the best known attribute at which girls excel is in linguistic ability, though curiously not in vocabulary. In my sample, girls scored equally with the boys on the Stanford–Binet vocabulary test. Although parents thought their sons were gifted twice as often as they did their daughters, there was no significant difference in the measured intelligence of either sex, in this particular sample.

Older boys are better at mathematical skills and at skills involving spatial relations (Garai and Scheinfeld, 1968). This can be seen in their relatively high scoring on the sub-test of the Wechsler Intelligence Scale for Children, called the 'Performance Scale', which measures practical and mathematical ability. Girls do relatively better on the 'Verbal Abilities' sub-scale. These levels of abilities appear to be stable characteristics of either sex, as they show up no matter which test is used. Clearly, using a test of verbal abilities or a maths test in school as an intelligence test would distort the results between boys and girls.

From the first word, girls show their linguistic ability. They speak earlier, read earlier, are better at English language and express themselves better; girls in my sample even had better handwriting. This superiority continues throughout school. Girls also learn to count earlier than boys and do as well as boys in arithmetic in primary school. But boys shoot ahead in early adolescence in their ability at arithmetical reasoning and spatial relations. Men continue this trend to show superiority in tasks which involve restructuring elements of a problem or the preliminary breakdown of established mental sets. This ability for categorization gives men a greater advantage in organizing or restructuring isolated events (Maccoby, 1966). Studies which find males superior in reasoning typically use experimental problems that, seeking to avoid the effects of past experience, ask the subject to juggle with the material being presented. This type of activity seems to suit the male mind, whereas female intuition is also reasoning, but of a different kind, being based on long-term experience, some of which may be forgotten or suppressed.

Since boys and girls have different rates and types of intellectual development, results on tests will be affected by the age at which they are measured. The future adult intelligence level of girls can be predicted between three and six years old, due to their speedy rate of intellectual growth during this time. However, boys' measurable intellectual growth takes place later – between six and ten years. During this later period, almost twice as many boys as girls show intellectual measurement increases (Kagan *et al.*, 1958). Terman *et al.* (1930) found that even though girls might decline in IQ during this period of the boys' growth, gifted girls achieved better marks than boys throughout their school years.

The measurement of IQ in boys and girls respectively is affected by the different rates at which they grow mentally; they will be able to do different things at different ages. Whereas the method of calculation of IQ involves a division of mental age by chronological age, the latter will remain constant for both sexes, but mental age will not. It is particularly notable on the Wechsler scale that girls' IQs begin to decline in late childhood, while those of boys increase. For girls, this indicates that their mental age results from items which have been accomplished for some time, while boys' rates of development are slower, later and possibly longer. These later types of development seem to be those of the 'male' computational abilities.

In spite of these demonstrated sex differences, there is considerable evidence showing that the most essential intellectual abilities for both sexes are verbal skills. The aspects of all intelligence tests which are the best predictors of the final score on the test are those of verbal ability. In America, verbal college aptitude scores are also the best predictors of college grades, as was true for the eleven-plus selection examination, which all British children took from 1945; it was the verbal scores in this that predicted outcomes best. Tests which avoid the verbal aspect – 'culture-free' tests – have proved to be less reliable or predictably valid than those which have verbal components, such as the Stanford–Binet. According to Goslin (1963), it is probable that verbal ability is of essential importance in the performance of virtually every task requiring high intelligence.

Vernon's cautionary words are worth quoting (Vernon *et al.*, 1977):

'Even where we find the greatest difference in abilities, the ratio of one sex to the other would be unlikely to exceed 60–40; in other words, if 60 males score above the general average in, say, maths, then 40 females do likewise. Similarly there might be 60 superior female spellers to 40 males. But at the gifted level (say the top 2 to 5 per cent) the odds become greater; probably at least three times as many boys as girls are likely to be specially talented in maths. However, there are no precise figures, and generalizations are dubious since we do not know enough about the effects of cultural pressures. On the whole, gifted children are less likely than non-gifted to be affected by these pressures. Thus very bright girls often show some conventionally masculine interests, and gifted boys show some feminine ones. In most respects, then, we may expect to find very much the same characteristics in gifted children of both sexes.'

## Creativity

In spite of concerted efforts to promote creativity in education and in industry, the concept remains ephemeral. There is argument as to whether it is an aspect of intelligence or independent of it. The term creative has most often been used of great artists or even great scientists, but of late it has come to take on more general, vaguely educational meanings such as in descriptions of toys or of the group experiences of sensitivity training. Where once it was considered to be the prerogative of a few gifted people, it is now seen as applying in some sense to all and especially to children. Everyone is seen to be creative, but their creativeness is not always apparent. This recent linguistic broadening of the concept of creativity is well nigh impossible to measure within our present technique. Present research work on creativity is a continued development of the original ideas of Guilford (1950).

American concentration on creativity in education is usually dated from the Russian success in the satellite race – Sputnik – in 1957. Lavish scholarship schemes were set up to encourage more science students to study the liberal arts, while educational psychologists carried the idea of divergent thinking into teacher training and into the classroom. Guilford's original tests were developed and used in a multitude of research studies. British efforts at stimulating creativity did not seem to have that 'take-off' impetus, but primary schools had for some time been promoting an imaginative approach to school work and, after all, we had not been in the race. Liam Hudson (1966) described the situation succinctly: 'Creativity . . . represents a boom in the American psychological industry, only paralleled by that of programmed learning'.

Although the creative gifted child is often considered to hold the greatest possible contribution to our civilization, this very child is the one most likely to slip through our educational and assessment net. Tests for creativity in all subjects are particularly bedevilled by subjectivity and unreliability. When different examiners assess the same scripts for creativity in, say, English, they often award widely differing marks. The advent of short-answer objective tests, now prevalent in American schools, has helped the reliability of marking but undercut the possibility of creative expression.

The value of a whole realm of mental faculties such as fluency, originability and flexibility was explained by Guilford (1950). He distinguished between types of thinking which he called 'convergent', where a child is expected to conform to what is already in the mind of the teacher, and 'divergent' thinking which is non-conforming and creative. His were the first tests of creativity in which the child had to suggest as many uses as he could for a brick, a newspaper and a tin can, or write down witty titles to stories, or devise different endings, or imagine what would happen if everyone doubled in height. Answers could readily be scored on the number of alternatives offered and on their rate of infrequency in the population. Some cynics regarded this as an invitation to the child to be silly. The tests and their statistical interpretation did expose mental ability factors which were relatively independent of other ability factors such as verbal. But it is very questionable whether the careful measurement of paper and pencil tests is comparable to the prolonged, concentrated application of technical expertise in creative endeavour.

Tests of divergent thinking have not been found to be reliably related to creativity in adults. But they have been found to distinguish between personality characteristics (MacKinnon, 1962). Highly creative children are often considered to be uninhibited in their thinking.

According to Hess and Shipman (1965), parents direct their children in two ways, which may be in 'imperatives' or 'instructives'. The 'imperative' is an unqualified command; the 'instructive' is information or a command which carries a justification. They consider the former to facilitate passive and compliant approaches by the child and the latter initiatory and assertive approaches which could lead to creative behaviour. Convergent and divergent styles of thinking are most probably linked to deeper differences in personality and attitudes.

Cattell (in Freeman *et al.*, 1968) has suggested that the creative person is, among other things, a 'self-sufficient introvert'. Like achievement motivation, success in creative effort has been associated with great encouragement to independence during childhood, whereas poor creative performance has been associated with dependence (Oden in Freeman *et al.*, 1968). In fact, creative effectiveness is probably governed by a similar essential element of risk-taking to that needed for achievement. There is a relationship between creativity and stability; an effectively creative child is sufficiently confident to be able to play and work freely without feeling the restrictions of what is 'right' and what is 'wrong'. He has acquired his own sturdy frame of reference, rather than being dependent on those of others. Effectively creative children are confident and have the freedom and security to take risks, to be curious and to be adventurous.

In a wider piece of research in which they attempted to separate the effects of intelligence and creative ability, Getzels and Jackson (1962) studied the mothers of children designated by their teachers as uncreative. The mothers were found to be vigilant about the 'correct' (according to external criteria) upbringing of their children. The authors suggested that permissive parents tend to grant their children a great deal of autonomy, allowing them to learn about the environment in their own terms, encouraging and rewarding their curiosity and independent behaviour. Parents who severely restrict their children's freedom may suppress their tendencies to explore and so inhibit their development towards independence. Thus undue restrictions, rather than leading to conformity and independent action, could heighten emotional tension which may express itself in rebellious, immature and emotionally unstable behaviour. An example of this behaviour pattern can be seen in the poet Sylvia Plath's letters to her mother, which have recently been published. It appears that her mother was very demanding and that her daughter, even at 30, was very dependent on her. The mother was the daughter's mirror in which she sought to shine – Sylvia even took her 'A' grades in the subjects that her mother had failed. She seemed to have a dependent need to constantly prove herself to her mother.

The work of Getzels and Jackson has been highly criticized on both design and statistical grounds, but their ideas have been seminal. A modified reproduction of their work with Scottish schoolchildren (Hasan and Butcher, 1966) found that intelligence and creativity scores overlapped so much that the results bore little resemblance to the parent study. They concluded that the atmosphere in the school was all-important. Torrance (1975) undertook 15 partial replications of the original study and found that 10 of them gave essentially the same results. Torrance too suggests that school atmosphere is essential to the encouragement of creative thinking abilities. Wallach and Kogan (1965) investigated creativity in primary school children; they tried to avoid brakes on creative activity such as anxiety, tiredness and verbal stimuli. By this means, they believed that they succeeded in separating creativity and intelligence, and it was concluded that highly creative children need a more relaxed school atmosphere than normal children.

From the evidence collected so far it would seem that the relationship between creativity and any other faculty, such as intelligence, is still very dependent on the nature of the investigation and on the measurement techniques employed. It is only possible to say with certainty that whereas a high IQ does not guarantee high creativity, a low IQ certainly militates against it. But the tests of divergent thinking have shown a relationship to a specific range of children's characteristics.

Highly divergent children make more contributions to classroom discussions, write more imaginative compositions, prefer less conventional friends and make more adventurous plans for the future. Those who score very highly on tests of intelligence but poorly on tests of creative thinking are particularly concerned with academic success and feel happier in a conventional structured school setting. Highly intelligent convergers tend to come from homes where there is pressure on them to succeed scholastically. Highly intelligent divergers come from homes which are less bound by concern for security and where the children are given much greater choice of friends and activities.

Torrance (1962 and 1965) has developed tests of creativity for use by teachers. His study of teachers' attitudes towards pupils showed that they had very mixed feelings about the highly creative child. Sadly, they appeared to value good manners, obedience and punctuality above courage in thought and action. He is particularly concerned to alert teachers to the identification and needs of creative children. A follow-up study by Torrance (1969) of children who were found to be very creative on his tests showed that in adulthood they appeared to lead more interesting, less static and more creative lives. He also claimed that female divergers bore less children. Perhaps this is one of the unrecognized forms of creativity which is decidedly convergent.

Tests for intelligence are recognizable for what they are, but tests for creativity are a relatively unknown measure. There is clearly a great deal of overlap and it might be considered that the addition of creativity tests to intelligence tests would aid in the discovery of gifted creators. But, because so much uncertainty still exists about it, there is no case for large-scale routine testing for creativity. Whilst investigatory testing is exciting and adding to the body of information all the time, the most promising leads in the study of creativity are concerned with development of children's characteristics in their social settings. Keeping children's minds open within an educational system is becoming an established goal in many parts of the world and the combined efforts of school and home are needed for this.

## ADJUSTMENT

The relationship between a child and his environment varies from day to day. Adjustment is never static; it is a learned form of behaviour, subject to the same principles that govern other forms of learning. This learned adjustment does affect other types of learning, such as school progress, whilst maladjustment is essentially a psycho-social concept, which overlaps but is not the same as delinquency. A child is termed maladjusted when his general adjustment to life is so poor that his unhappiness deflects his development from its expected route. Such children can show their adverse condition in many ways, which are not necessarily anti-social. Delinquency, on the other hand, is the term used when an offence has been committed.

Everyone has periods of maladjustment, such as depression after influenza or aggression due to fatigue and frustration. On the whole, these brief troubled times are recognized as episodes that will pass, but potential long-term maladjustment needs to be carefully examined before any official interfering action is taken. Many children's 'behaviour disorders', such as bedwetting or fear of the dark, will disappear simply with the passage of time.

The difference between a problem child and a 'normal' child is quantitative not qualitative. In other words, a problem arises when other people involved with the child find her behaviour to be less than tolerable. Clearly, children with socially acceptable behaviour will not be sent for professional attention because of their behaviour. Only those children whose behaviour is recognized as being a problem will invoke intervention on the part of an adult.

The word 'normal' is used in two different ways and it is necessary to distinguish between them:

*Statistical normality* is what characterizes the majority of the population. It is an average or norm. Usually, the top or bottom 3% of a range of behaviour is considered to be abnormal. This terminology would be used, for example in a survey of the heights of children of a given age. It is also used to identify gifted children.

*Ideal normality* is what we believe is normal or should be normal – in the sense of being problem-free, but this is not always with reference to actual reality, though. For example, continuous good health is regarded as ideally normal, whereas it is statistically abnormal. By the same token, a bright, good-looking healthy child is ideally normal, but the statistically average or 'normal' child has only an average amount of these qualities.

For the researcher, that which is normal in either sense can only be related to the society in which the study is carried out. Even within one society, what is considered to be normal varies over a period of time. For example, because of the new concept ideas of teaching, mathematical tables are not always taught by rote, as they used to be in primary schools in Britain. Consequently, measures of mathematical ability devised several years ago, which extract this kind of information, will show a fall in 'mathematical ability'. New methods of education are then decried as being less good than the old ones. But, in truth, we need new tests all the time to measure new styles of learning, in order to say what is normal for now. The effect of change over time makes comparison between old and new systems of any aspect of behaviour very difficult, if not impossible. Every generation of adults remembers that children were better behaved in their own childhood; it is not always easy to accept that all definitions of normality are relative.

In terms of children's behaviour and adjustment, local patterns can vary, even from family to family. In a conventional school, where children are obliged to remain seated and silent for most of the day, such behaviour is regarded as statistically and ideally normal. In an open-plan, child-centred school the child who remained seated and silent all day would be regarded as withdrawn and abnormal.

Normality must also be seen in terms of the child's own age. First-time parents are often very upset when their child begins to change his behaviour pattern, such as throwing tantrums at two years old. It is not unusual for a two-year-old to have a tantrum, but it is abnormal at eleven years old.

## Behaviour disorders

Michael Rutter, the eminent child psychiatrist, put forward two principles by which one might recognize and classify child behaviour disorders (Rutter, 1965). Firstly, recognition must be based on facts – what the child actually does. This operational first principle must take into account how frequently this behaviour occurs and in what context. Secondly, to be of use, the category must convey a description of relevant behaviour and carry some predictive value. To say that a child is naughty or mischievous fulfills neither of these categories.

Gifted children are often described as needing less sleep than other children. An original experiment was conducted into factors affecting the development of intelligence in infancy by Lawson and Ingleby (1974), who observed the daily routines of 54 families. They found that the amount of measured sleep decreased steadily with age, but that the second-born child was put to bed more often during the day, and actually slept more than the first-born child. The varying range of time during which infants were expected to sleep was considerable. Waking up was expected from 6.00 to 10.30 a.m. and going to sleep from 5.30 to 11 p.m. Wakefulness during the night also decreased with age. Higher social class infants both slept longer and woke and went to sleep earlier than lower class infants. As I found myself (Chapter 4) sleep was not a function of giftedness, but of social expectation.

The two primary groups of problems of maladjustment in children are neurotic disorders and anti-social or conduct disorders (Rutter,

1965). These correspond with the two types of disorder described by Stott (1976), whose technique was used to categorize the behaviour of my research sample. He called them under- and over-reaction (Chapter 4).

Stott believes that his adjustment guides could be used regularly in schools in a simplified form to assist teachers in spotting children who are high risks. The idea of screening for psychological maladjustment in schools, just as we screen for medical problems, is repugnant to many people, which is probably why these easily administered, well validated and easily accessible measures have never been used as intended. Innumerable children are therefore free to progress from maladjustment to delinquency, unhampered by psychologists. But the general fear in the Western world of authorized social control will probably be sufficient to keep assessment for maladjustment at bay for the foreseeable future.

## Sources of maladjustment

A highly informative study was carried out in California by Love and Kaswan (1974) which compared the environments of children who were seen as 'disturbed' by their teachers and of a matched group of 'normal' children. The research design was very similar to my own (Chapter 4), which compared the environments of children seen as gifted by their parents with those of a matched group of normal children.

Love and Kaswan recognized early on that their own professional values of behaviour were unrealistic and too simple. They found that the children who were mostly at risk of disturbed behaviour were those for whom adult behaviour was complex and confusing. Such a child is unable to distinguish appropriate from inappropriate cues as to what to do, and cannot therefore be clear and constructive in his responses to them. Information feedback, particularly in the form of videotapes of adult–child interaction played back to the families, was often immediately informative and effective in bringing about easier flowing relationships.

Their primary discovery – that the confusion of messages in adult–child communication is highly influential in the form and development of maladjustment – is in accord with the findings of many other studies (e.g. Peterson *et al.*, 1959; Winter and Ferreira, 1969; Zax and Cowen, 1969).

Unfortunately, Love and Kaswan decided that because home circumstances were so varied, they would bring the parents and children into a clinical setting (necessarily artificial) to watch their interaction. This was a strange decision in view of the prime objectives of the research, i.e. to see children in their natural environments, and must throw some doubt on the value of their report. They also had so few girls in their sample that any comparison between attitudes and behaviours of the two sexes was statistically impossible, which is a pity.

They found in the school situation, however, that teacher and parent behaviour patterns in conjunction contributed significantly towards the child's specific response at school. The researchers concluded that teachers, like parents, have too little expertise in recognizing those characteristics of both verbal and non-verbal behaviour in children which cause them distress. In brief, they found, as I did myself, that the child's 'ongoing interpersonal environment' is critical for his social effectiveness, at least as manifested in the school setting. The quality of the home background, then, is the all-important difference between those children who are recognized as troubled and those who are seen as normal in school.

Maladjustment in gifted children may be judged by their poor achievement in school. Another method which was used by Grotberg (1975) involved adults who had become patients in a mental hospital. They were, for that reason, regarded as under-achievers or failures as adults by the researchers. She studied 40 gifted adults who had an IQ range of 120–137 and compared them with normal adults of a 80–100 IQ range; they were of both sexes. None of the gifted group would have been called by that term in educational studies, as their IQ range was insufficiently high and 'gifted' seems to be a strong word to use of people in that IQ range, though some interesting results were reported in comparing the two groups. The gifted maladjusted under-achiever still felt superior, particularly the men, but even so, the gifted group nearly all saw themselves as failures – more than the non-gifted group. The gifted positively did not like work; they reported excessive conflicts with their parents (especially the men) and more than the non-gifted had shown an attempt to do better than their parents had done. Even at this level of intellectual ability, there seemed to have been a threat of failure hanging over the gifted group during childhood. It would have been a much more informative study had the researchers been able to find out what sort of pressure and expectation the subjects had been under during their lives. Were they in fact different to those of other non-institutionalized gifted adults?

Further discussion of stress and its consequences in the home environment was presented in Chapter 2.

## Stress in school

All children, whether gifted or not, are very vulnerable – at the mercy of adverse social influences and personal pressures. Both school and home can be painful and even permanently damaging experiences. But individual children will react to them differently, according to their particular qualities and their ages. In school, children are obliged to readjust continually to new teachers and every so often to a new school system. The achievement which a child shows in school may be closely related to the style of teaching of a particular teacher. If so, then a change of teachers is likely to mean a change in the pupil's achievement level. Adjustment and development at home and school always represent a process of interaction.

Schools have their own specialities of stress production. 'The pressures of mark-obsessed teachers (backed up by over-keen parents) can frequently be seen to produce irritability, jealousy between classmates, psychosomatic disorders and sheer fatigue' (Mays, 1973). Parents who are ambitious for their children realize that, because examination success is essential for further educational progress, they cannot afford to relax and allow their children to develop at their own pace. It is only children from non-aspiring homes who can be permitted to regard learning as a pleasure.

Strain and tension, brought about by a formal, ambitious educational system, can produce the symptoms of maladjustment in children who are already stress-prone or emotionally disturbed. This vulnerability may either be because of their family backgrounds or because of innate disposition. But schools themselves are often to blame for pupils' maladaptation; the more control a school exerts, the less concern is usually shown for the individual pupil and his self-concept. Strict control appears to exist in order to promote learning, but, in excess, it can act against it. Children who cannot accept the values of the school as relevant to their lives may 'drop out', either mentally or physically, and will then show their feelings in maladjusted behaviour.

Educational systems in industrial societies are sometimes considered as having a bias against mental good health. The effectiveness of schools is measured in terms of productivity rather than quality. Gestures are made in the direction of such attributes as caring, imagination, resourcefulness, co-operation and commitment, but not the specific teaching of them. Bronfenbrenner (1974) compared American schools, which he considered to be individualistic and competitive, with Russian schools with their provision for co-operative activities. He found that American children's experiences reinforced their sense of isolation and consequently increased hostility to their peers and the outside world. He saw their schools as drilling information into children, rather than helping to evolve rounded, productive members of society.

Bronfenbrenner believes that American schools should be re-integrated into the community, with children of different ages working together in responsible involvement, inside and outside school. Russian schools have a pattern of 'group adoption', through which each class takes the responsibility for the care of a group of younger children, possibly outside the school in a kindergarten. Similar moves to give children responsibility for others are growing in the United States, while schools which cater for all ages of children and adult scholars, called Community Schools, are becoming more frequent in Britain. This kind of school is designed to serve the community so that anyone may join in, whatever their age; there is active community involvement, not restricted to conventional school hours. As these schools are new and serve such a wide variety of people, they are particularly well equipped and staffed. However, we will have to wait and see whether the children who emerge from them are different in outlook and behaviour from their contemporaries in more conventional schools.

Teachers are not angels; favouritism and vindictiveness are well known in the classroom – behaviour which can only stem from the teachers' own unhappiness. But their effects on children are not well researched; the same child may be picked on independently by several teachers in different lessons, or for great lengths of time by one teacher. The gifted child may frequently be told at school how much is expected of him; added to his parents' explicit high expectations, the burden of being gifted may then become intolerable. Parents of gifted children often say that their children are more subject to ridicule, and to having their efforts deflated with sarcasm than other children in the class. If the learning experience is unpleasant or biased against them, any child may under-achieve, hate the daily torment and misbehave, no less the gifted child.

Above all teaching is a social task, though teachers are never chosen for their sensitivity in social relations. Consequently, there are teachers in positions of great authority over children who are quite unsuitable for their work. There is no system of social vetting of teachers anywhere, either before appointment or during their tenure of posts. Both bad teaching and bad social relationships inflict misery on innumerable children. School counsellors may help to alleviate the distress, though many American counsellors are overly concerned with programming timetables and British school counsellors are still few and far between.

## The development of hostility

Aggressive or hostile behaviour in children, particularly in boys, is considered by some theorists to be instinctive. Familiar hypotheses, such as the Oedipus and castration complexes and the death wish are part of the essence of Freudian theory. Lorenz (1966) and his followers in the ethological school claim that aggression and wars are 'natural'.

These ideas are evolved from a society based on competition – a close relative of aggression. Many longitudinal studies of aggression have shown this connection (Kagan and Moss, 1962; Nelson *et al.*, 1969). The schools in which children spend a third of their lives are themselves reflections of the society around them in that they accept a competitive system and an individualistic ethos. They have been seen in growing research findings to be active agents, rather than passive witnesses to the process of selection and allocation of pupils for their future social and economic roles.

The intensive work of Hargreaves in England (1967, and Hargreaves *et al.*, 1975) has shown how schools operate over time to divide the pupils from one another and instil hostile attitudes between different groups. He found that the primary causes of this school-induced hostility were rigid streaming, strongly held academic objectives and an inflexible and often authoritarian structure. Unfortunately, as with much research evidence, Hargreaves only studied boys' schools. There is practically no information available on social relationships and maladjustment in girls' schools and little comparable evidence from English mixed schools. We cannot assume that they will be the same.

Aggression is being viewed more and more as a learned rather than an inborn behaviour (Selg, 1975). It is considered to develop from birth onwards as the baby discovers the value of insistent hostility as a means of getting what it wants. Crying loudly or screaming normally brings food and comfort, though children also copy aggressive habits from adults. Child rearing patterns and parent and teacher examples of behaviour are together of supreme importance in the children's learning of aggression through identification.

There is considerable evidence that aggressive parents tend to have aggressive children (Bandura and Walters, 1963). Children who were exposed to aggressive adult models were found to be significantly more aggressive themselves, when exposed to frustration, than children exposed to non-aggressive adult models. This imitative behaviour in children is strengthened by continued reinforcement, which in practice is all too frequently available. Were there to be a change in the behaviour of adults, we could expect a change in the behaviour of children. Margaret Mead has demonstrated in her studies of non-Western peoples that a non-aggressive culture continues to produce passive behaviour in adults and children.

Intensive success in achievement can only be obtained with the use of aggression of a specific sort. I discovered in my research (Chapter 4) that successful, ambitious parents of children whom they believed to be gifted tended to produce ambitious offspring. These aspiring children were seen by their teachers as significantly more hostile than their peers. They appeared to be less well adjusted to their social environments, both of home and school. Because of this, some of them were probably reacting badly to pressures on them and were actually doing less well than would have been expected at school. Hostility can be a two-edged sword.

## Seeking help

Some children use a pretence of maladjustment as a means of avoiding unpleasant issues, such as demands for harder work or challenges. Adults usually understand these deviations for what they are. Outside help is normally sought only when the child's behaviour reaches such a level that the adults concerned feel they can no longer cope. The spectrum of available help ranges from friends, via voluntary lay societies of other people with the same problem, to professionals. The parents and teachers of troubled gifted children have their own societies, to which they may turn for help, in several countries. As gifted children are necessarily exceptional by virtue of their ability, it could be expected that adults seeking assistance would put this most obvious reason forward as the cause of any disturbance that may be present in the child.

Children recognized as maladjusted will usually be seen at a child guidance clinic, where they may be given some form of psychotherapy. The psycho-analytical type of treatment has been found to be of limited effectiveness, except possibly with some forms of interpersonal difficulties. Its availability, in Britain at least, is also very restricted.

*128*

Behaviour modification techniques are now used more frequently and parents and teachers are brought into the therapeutic programme. Through these techniques, children are taught to develop new behavioural patterns.

Problem behaviour in the normal child, that is the child who is not psychiatrically ill, is considered in terms of behaviour modification to be caused by the child having learned the wrong responses. It is also believed that what has been learned can be unlearned. Inefficient and confused communication are considered to be prime causes of mislearning. Treatment is devised in terms of the environmental effects which are maintaining the child's maladjusted behaviour, rather than of possible past causes. Different problems appear at characteristically different ages.

During treatment, parents are shown how their own behaviour can influence their child's behaviour. They are taught how to build up an appropriate repertoire of desired behaviours in basic stages. These new behaviours are reinforced by attention from adults, while unwelcome behaviour is ignored and discouraged by such actions as leaving the room during a display of temper. Everything is explained to the child in its simplest form and long in-depth discussion is positively avoided. Rewards and praise are used plentifully and the tasks are gradually increased in complexity.

The need for consistency in a behaviour modification programme of therapy is crucial. All the adults involved, as well as the child, should know what is going on; this means grandparents and teachers too. Maladaptive behaviour often increases at first because the child anticipates a breakdown in consistency. This method needs time to work and a daily record of progress usually gives encouragement to parents. Gifted children are particularly good at spotting parents' maximum areas of vulnerability, and they aim at them. But gifted children are just as amenable as others to the satisfaction of praise, rewards, clear instruction and appropriate expectation of behaviour.

# CHAPTER 4

# The Gulbenkian Project on Gifted Children

There is no possibility at present – and it is unlikely that there ever will be – of placing a child at a point on a spectrum of giftedness. It would make research very much easier to be able to say that Belinda is 90% able in arithmetic or that Bill is in the top 2% of social ability. But in fact, as educational psychology stands at present, it is not possible to make a precise measure of the individual gifts of a child over a range of possible abilities. Standardized tests in specific subjects such as mathematics or geography do exist of course, but a child can only be judged in comparison to others with the same educational experience and the same preparation for that style of testing. There are tests in America designed to measure progress at the end of each grade year, but again these are not always interchangeable even between states, and certainly not between cultures. In addition, to be gifted usually implies that the child is over the top of the scale and is thus, by definition, unmeasurable by that particular instrument.

The Gulbenkian research was based on the definition made by parents that their children were outstanding in some way. It is important to note that the children were not accepted into the research as having been measured as gifted, but as being seen as gifted by their parents. They could therefore be called 'designated' gifted children; at the start of the research their real abilities were unknown. They were to be compared with children who were not described as gifted by their parents.

By comparing children whose parents believed them to be gifted with children whose parents did not, it was hoped that the reasons would emerge why the parents had taken these decisions. The sample of parents who believed their children to be gifted was available from the records of the National Association for Gifted Children.

# SETTING UP THE PROJECT

The preliminary source of children was the collection of correspondence which had accumulated in the offices of the National Association for Gifted Children (NAGC) between 1966 and 1974, just prior to the start of the enquiry. The NAGC is a registered charity which anyone – parents, local authorities, psychiatrists etc. – may contact on behalf of a child whom they consider may be gifted. There are branches of the Association all over Great Britain; a few branches demand proof of some ability in a child, but most do not. The Association provides Saturday activities, special lectures and camps for 'gifted' children; it also provides a counselling service and fees are very low.

The accumulated records were in a wide variety of uncategorized forms. They were sometimes letters of enquiry from interested persons, headteachers' reports, or detailed case histories from child guidance clinics. The correspondence was from all over the British Isles.

The first task was to categorize this information so that a workable experimental sample of children might be extracted from it. There were in fact about 6500 sets of correspondence concerning about 4500 children. The information was all placed on punched record cards; only when this task was complete was it possible to begin the sampling process.

## Selecting the target group

This first group of children, selected from the records of the NAGC were known as the target group, T. The criteria by which they were selected were as follows:

(1)    One parent had at some time been a member of NAGC within the years 1971–74.

(2)    The child lived and went to school within the geographical North West of England.

(3)    The child was in the statutory school attendance age-range, i.e. 5 to 16 years old.

The target group was thus defined by time (recency), geography (North West) and age (5–16 years). There were 112 children fulfilling these criteria. A letter was sent to all the families in this target sample, outlining the research and asking them if they would participate. There were several reasons why some of this original sample did not take part in the research; these were the conventional ones, such as removal from the area, accidents or refusal to participate.

## Selecting the control groups

When the parents of the T group had given their agreement to involvement in the research, the child's school was asked to participate. This proved to be a complicated process, as a number of the parents were loath to tell the headteachers about their membership of the NAGC. They said they feared the head might feel his authority was threatened, that he might think they were over-doting parents, that he might treat their child unfairly from then on or that, in general, this knowledge of their behaviour would spoil their 'good' relationship with the head.

Many parents agreed to participate only if they could tell or ask the headteachers first. Some gave specific instructions, such as 'don't write, phone first' or 'she'll like you if you speak with a posh accent' or 'try him through the priest'.

It was essential to have the schools' co-operation in this research, both to fill in the total picture of the child's environment and to help in selecting the control children. The majority of headteachers were in agreement. But the situation in Britain is that headteachers do have considerable power in their own schools. They can refuse entry if they wish and have been known to do so, both to parents and to researchers. Those children whose schools refused to participate had to be dropped from the project, even though their parents were willing to participate. The whole school class of each of the target group children was screened, using the Raven's Matrices test (Raven, 1965). Two control children were selected for each target child from the screening data.

## The first control group – $C_1$

These were children matched with the target group for ability, age, sex and school class. The essential difference between them and the target group was that their parents were not members of the NAGC; the most important similarity was in their measured intellectual ability. The parents and children who were selected by the screening were then asked to take part in the research.

# The second control group – $C_2$

These were children, chosen at random from the same school class and matched only for age and sex. They were similar to the other two groups in having the same educational experience and being drawn from the same school catchment area, but were different in that their intellectual ability was disregarded. In that respect, they were chosen at random; they too were asked to take part in the research.

Selecting the second control group in this way could give rise to two difficulties. Firstly, that the class was not 'normal' – it could be preselected by the wealth of the parents or the children's ability, in a selective school. This control group would not then be a 'normal' control, representative of British children. Secondly, children could be part of this control group, but, by being randomly selected on ability, could turn out to be gifted. This could have the effect of blurring the comparisons between the groups. However, with these and other cautions in mind, the three groups described above formed the basis of the research.

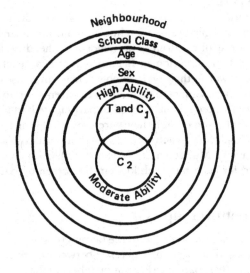

*Matching the experimental groups*

There were now three groups of children, who were matched on school catchment area, educational experience, age and sex. The target and first control group were also matched on intellectual ability and the two control groups on non-membership of the NAGC. The target group was the only one whose parents had presented them as gifted.

The final number of children in each of the three groups was 70, providing a sample of 210 children. Their ages were from 5 to 14 years, the distribution of their ages resembling a normal curve exactly – which was purely fortuitous. They went to 61 schools, of all types. These were 48 non-denominational schools, seven Roman Catholic, four Church of England and two Jewish schools. Thirty-nine per cent of the schools were private, compared to the national average of about 3%. Over all the areas covered, there was a heterogeneous class structure, which presented a wide variety of life styles. Virtually all the children in the sample were in fact white and of English descent, but absolutely no discrimination as to race was intended.

## Design

In the realms of social science, nothing is cut and dried; things are not always as they seem. Unconscious preconceptions get in the way and it is impossible to take a unified, truly scientific approach. Because of the variety of material to be gathered in this research, a variety of methods were used; they were all intended to be interrelated and to be contained within a framework of theory. But the design did allow for recognized subjective techniques.

Primarily, each child was regarded as an individual, rather than a statistic. This involved a greater familiarity with the children and their families than is perhaps usual in educational 'field' research. Homes and schools were visited more than once for each child and the investigator was thus better able to get to know the people involved. This familiarity added greatly to the richness of the material assembled.

Every child completed a battery of tests which, depending on their quickness, took up to about four hours to complete. This took place during several sessions; the tests are described below. The children were also given a questionnaire about their interests and outlook on life.

All the parents were interviewed at home, using a pre-rated questionnaire of 90 items. This was intended both as a guide for the interviewer and as a means of facilitating responses. Ten aspects of the home background were also assessed by the interviewer and recorded on the questionnaire.

The headteachers were interviewed with a pre-rated questionnaire of 40 questions. Class teachers filled in the Stott Social Adjustment Guide (Stott, 1976) for each of the three children taking part in the research, from the same school class. The school was also assessed by the interviewer and recorded on the questionnaire.

## The comparisons

Three major comparisons formed the greater part of the statistical investigation of the data which had been obtained in homes and schools.

(a) *The experimental groups* – The original aim of the research had been to investigate whether there were any notable relationships in respect of behaviour or ability between the target and control groups. Each of these groups was compared with the other two on all aspects of the information.

(b) *The IQ groups* – When this first comparison had been made, all the children were exempted from their original groups and, regardless of the group they had been in before, were reassigned to two new groups. One was composed of high IQ children, who had been measured on the Stanford–Binet intelligence test as having an IQ of 141 or more. The other was a moderate IQ group, containing children who had a measured IQ of 140 or less on the same test. These two groups were then compared on all the same parameters. The purpose was to find out if measured intelligence alone could be found to have behavioural effects, irrespective of parents' beliefs.

(c) *The adjustment groups* – The children were again re-sorted and placed into groups, which were formed by their scores on the Bristol Social Adjustment Guides (BSAG). This was the measure of how the teachers perceived the children's behaviour in the classroom. There were three groups – of high, moderate and low BSAG scores; the groups were compared with each other on all parameters. By this move, it was intended to disentangle the children's observed behaviour in school from their abilities and home influences.

## Measures used in the project

The screening measure for intellectual ability was the Raven's Progressive Matrices, followed by the individually presented Stanford–Binet intelligence test. A description of these tests and of the reasons why they were chosen for this project are given on page 104.

## The personality questionnaires

All the personality measures used were variations of the ones prepared in Illinois, USA, based on a statistical analysis of data about personality which have been collected over thousands of children for many years (Cattell and Cattell, 1973; Coan and Cattell, 1976; Porter and Cattell, 1959).

Cattell divides observed behaviour into traits. Between 16 and 21 traits have been identified for different groups of people and different collections of them are used in the questionnaire. For example, the adult personality questionnaire (the 16PF), uses 16 traits, but the children's personality questionnaire (CPQ) uses only 14 of them. Each of these traits is relatively independent of the others, so that although a child may occupy a given position along one dimension, it will not necessarily affect her position on another. The traits which were selected as a basis of comparison in this research were those which all the age-groups had in common.

Although research on these questionnaires is extensive, the subjects were all American. When the adult questionnaire was re-standardized on British subjects recently, a number of widely different norms were found between results from the two cultures. Clearly, British children do not live in an identical culture to American children and the test has not been re-standardized for them. Not only are their life styles and expectations different, but there are notable language confusions. The less Americanized a British child is, the less he will comprehend 'act rude', 'big bug', 'get mad', etc. However, as comparisons in this project were only made between groups of English children, it is unlikely that the subtle gradations of American awareness between them would have had a pronounced effect on the results.

A degree of caution is always necessary in generalizing from any one body of work, such as that of Cattell. The traits isolated in the analysis of his data will obviously depend for their value on the original measures which he chose to use. However, there was a possibility that personality profiles obtained by using these detailed questionnaires might distinguish between gifted and less able children. If intellectual ability was found to be highly related to personality traits, the identification of gifted children would be assisted. Those who say that gifted children have different personalities from normal children would then be vindicated.

## The music practical test

It was only because of their children's intellectual or musical ability that this sample of parents had joined the National Association for Gifted Children. Other specific abilities were clearly held to be of less importance. Even other scholastic abilities, such as mathematics or language, were not presented as reasons for the definition of 'gifted' by parents. Four target children and eight control children attended a school for the musically gifted.

In order to test musical ability, a specially designed test, used in previous research to distinguish musically talented children was used (Freeman, 1974). The assumption was that the musically talented should be able to reproduce a known tune, played by unfamiliar means, more quickly than the non-talented.

In order to avoid the effect of practice and tuition, an experimental instrument was devised, which was novel to each child, yet simple enough to play at once. The result was a set of individual chime-bars; each one gives a specified note when tapped with a stick. A simple, familiar tune of seven notes was chosen and was presented to each child in a predetermined wrong order. She would then be timed in putting the bars into the correct order, but, as some children could not complete the task at all, a time limit of three minutes was set.

## The Bristol Social Adjustment Guides

This measure of the social adjustment of children in school has been developed by Stott in Ontario for over 20 years. The day school edition is concerned with how children are seen by their teachers to behave in class. 'It provides a means of detecting and assessing behaviour disturbances (maladjustment) in children aged five to sixteen years within a school setting' (Stott, 1976). The teacher reports factually on what is observed. 'Behaviour which may be unacceptable to the teacher, or which may appear unusual only because of cultural differences, is disregarded.' A four-page booklet of 250 descriptions of behaviour is given to the teacher, who underlines those which apply to the child being assessed. The coded items then provide a numerical picture of the child's adjustment in school.

There are two main scales of maladjustment – Under-reaction and Over-reaction. These are composed of sub-sections, which can be used independently as measures of, for example, peer maladaptiveness or distractability. The higher the score, the more indications there are of deviant behaviour. Research on the day school edition by the National Child Development Study in England (Davie *et al.*, 1972) has shown some consistency between the scores of the sexes, but boys are found much more frequently to be over-reactive and especially inconsequential. This means that they are more likely to act first and think later. There were virtually no differences between the different age levels.

Socio-economic differences were more pronounced in the English study than in Stott's Canadian research, the lower social classes scoring more highly on maladjustment in England. However, rural children, although of lower class, did show less maladjusted behaviour than city children. This was confirmed by Rutter *et al.* (1974), who found a much higher rate of maladjustment among children in Inner London than among those in the Isle of Wight. Both the Canadian and English studies found that physically unhealthy and later-born children were more prone to behaviour disturbance than other children.

## The parents' questionnaire

The interview with the parents was designed as a descriptive and numerical measure of parental attitudes and of the children's home backgrounds. It included personal details of both parents, such as occupation and education, their attitudes to education and their descriptions of the children. Although memory can play tricks in, say, describing a child's first words, all three experimental groups of target and control children were subject to the same process in this respect. It was what the parents believed that was important in this study. If, for example, the children were seen by one group of parents to be more alert at birth than the other groups, this belief could be compared with other parental beliefs and (in some respects) with the child's measured behaviour.

A pre-rated assessment of the home and surrounding environment was carried out for each family. The main aim of this aspect of the investigation was to quantify the kind of encouragement and opportunity which the children found at home. At least one visit was made to each of the 210 homes.

# The children's questionnaire

The children were asked about their interests and activities, what they wanted to do in life and what they thought was expected of them. They were asked how they approached a task and how they felt about their relationships with other people; of particular importance were the questions which referred to their thinking processes. This questionnaire was intended as a measure of the children's perception of life. Did gifted children see life differently from other children and how were they affected by their parents' views of them?

# The headteachers' questionnaire

In addition to the Social Adjustment Guide, which the class teachers completed, the headteacher of each school was interviewed. The questionnaire was designed to find out the headteachers' attitudes to education, especially with regard to gifted children. On the whole, the way a school is run is closely related to the aims of the headteacher. The simplest way to find out about the schools in this sample was to ask their heads.

## Collecting the data

The practical aspects of research are, of course, as important as the theoretical ones. As this was a three-directional approach to the children in their social context, the means by which the data were collected are described in that way.

# The parents

The first research contacts were with the parents of the target sample – those who had joined the National Association for Gifted Children. Apart from the loss of parents from the research for technical reasons such as moving house, the parents often gave personal reasons, some of which are offered below.

'We think because of the attitudes at his school, it would not be of benefit to our son.'

Mother worried that the school would use his involvement in the project 'against him'. He had 'enough' problems already at school, where his ability went unrecognized.

'Owing to current domestic circumstances, we would prefer it if Jane were not involved at present.'

Straight refusal with no reasons, but information on the case suggested that the boy is at a school for the maladjusted.

Only son, sent to boarding school out of research area, because day education was 'insufficient for a child with his superior abilities'.

Absolute refusal, no logical reasons offered, but mother said that 'the school wouldn't like it'.

Refused because on a previous occasion child had had his name splashed all over a popular newspaper, although the interviewer concerned agreed to keep the child's name secret.

Boy refused. Mother said it was due to problems over father's death and would not attempt to persuade him, viz: 'At this present time, neither Martin nor ourselves wish him to be involved in a project of this kind. We feel that he is coping with sufficient involvement in life at a boarding school, and consider that he should not be subject to any additional test.'

Contact with the control children's parents had the blessing of the school to support it. The letter which the control groups' parents received did not mention the NAGC. As the control parents were not members of this organization, it was judged that their answers to the questionnaire would be less likely to be biased, if the word 'gifted' were avoided. It was not considered to be good interview procedure that such a laden concept should be given as the main reason for the research. It was hoped that, by this means, control parents would not respond to the questions either towards or away from 'giftedness', as it affected them. The project was termed 'The Gulbenkian Project' after its benefactor and parents were told that it was a survey into child development.

The interviews all took place in the parents' homes. Depending more on the parent than the interviewer, the length of time taken varied from about one to two hours. The loneliness of housewives was probably the most frequent cause of a long interview. Sometimes the rest of the family were present, even though one specific child was being talked about; this probably affected the level of intimacy during the interview, but was unavoidable. Some parents demanded considerable detail of the research plan at the doorstep (even with the known approval of the school and the University), before they would agree to be questioned.

Others made strenuous efforts to be available for the interview, one family even returning from holiday early. As the triad of children were at the same school, the control parents were occasionally aware by means of the school grapevine that something was going on before they were approached. Several parents contacted the research base to ask why they had been left out.

Home environments varied from large houses in their own grounds to poor, unkempt terraced housing. Interiors were occasionally very imaginative. One tiny terraced house was decorated inside like a night-club; the walls of the front room were dark, with heavy velvet curtains and plastic/leather furniture. The mother explained that they were 'show-people'. Another council house was like a showroom with almost no furniture, but contained lighted glass cases of live members of the reptile family, including a huge iguana in its own show-case. There were also tin soldiers and Victoriana, lit up on display. Such visual drama was not, however, usual.

## The school

Most of the teachers replied to the introductory letter, but a few had to be contacted by telephone. Reasons for refusal varied between lack of time, space and, by implication, energy. A few interesting quotations from headteachers are given below.

'I do feel that we must take care not to involve the girls too frequently in research of various kinds.'

'We have so many demands of this kind.'

'High ability children. Although I must agree that there is some need for investigation into this aspect of education, I do not at present consider it high enough on my present priorities to offer the facilities you require.'

One headteacher was angry that the target parents had been approached without his permission. He felt that it was a matter for him, as a caring headmaster, to decide whether one of his children entered a research project or not. Parents could not be expected to make informed judgements of that kind. Naturally, he refused access to the school. Another headmaster insisted that an explanation of the project be delivered to him in person and not by telephone or letter. His refusal, after this obeisance, was delivered promptly.

*142*

Refusals were almost entirely from primary school headmasters. The heads of other, apparently more 'important', schools could not have been more helpful. In many primary schools, particularly infant ones, teachers forsook their classes and helped in using the screening procedure. The teachers and children most often appeared to enjoy the short break in their everyday activities. Class teachers were also very willing and prompt in filling in the Social Adjustment inventory for their three pupils. All the headteachers who agreed to participate filled in the questionnaire designed for the project.

## The children

Every child was asked if he or she would take part in the project since unwilling participation would probably have a lowering effect on test results. Considerable effort went into making the children mentally comfortable and, as most of the testing was carried out in the child's home, it was usually successful. In this way, it is probable that the results of the intelligence test and children's questionnaire were about as accurate a reflection of the children's abilities and attitudes as it is possible to obtain. Generally, the children were delighted to receive this unusual amount of attention and did their best to do as requested.

Subjectively, the children of extremely high IQ were very impressive to the interviewer. They seemed to have a dry sense of humour, which was used only occasionally in what appeared to be a very serious world. They were also physically very attractive, sure of themselves, and looked about with a particularly direct gaze. But they did not ask a multitude of questions, nor show very much curiosity about the research project.

## THE EXPERIMENTAL GROUPS

The collected material amounted to 217 pieces of data or variables. There were 210 children to be examined and compared on each of them. The matrix of data was very large and had therefore to be clearly organized. All the data were subjected to the same type of measurements and statistical analysis. These were primarily factor analysis and analysis of variance, but other methods of interpretation were also used.

The first interpretive act was to examine as a whole all the data from all the children, their families and schools. This was to see what sort of a sample it was, and whether there were any notable relationships between the variables. The first impression from this examination was that the sample was largely a collection of high social-class, well-educated families. Both fathers' and mothers' occupations and educational levels were high, as had been those of the child's grandparents before them. Most of the families lived in good accommodation, in a good neighbourhood. The parents read high quality newspapers and had a much higher than average number of books in their homes.

Many of the children had been to nursery school and they were often described by their parents as bright and independent, though emotional and highly strung. There was much more hostility and generally difficult behaviour in the children than could have been expected from a sample of normal children. There was also an element of unhappiness, if not depression, among the sample children.

As parents in this relatively high social bracket had been able to exercise much more choice in their selection of school than is usual, it was important to find out what kind of schools the children went to. Not all the schools had been chosen or even approved of by the parents, but every school concerned had at least one child whose parents believed her to be gifted. The schools had come into the research by virtue of having a target group child in their ranks, and the two control children had been selected from the school class.

The picture of the headteacher which emerged was that of a sympathetic person who is concerned to do the best for his pupils' development. In this sample, 84% of the children were below secondary school age (about 11 years) which may have accounted for the considerable concern headteachers showed for general child development, rather than academic achievement. The headteachers of the 61 schools were very varied in their attitudes to education. On the whole, they did not consider the gifted child to be a problem, but were sympathetic to possible difficulties. Headteachers did not appear to be concerned with the social class of their pupils; they believed rather that a child's positive attitude to education was all-important.

## The target and control groups

First investigations into the experimental groups showed that the target parents seemed to take their children's education more seriously than the control parents. They seemed to have tried particularly hard to give their children the best possible educational start in life, with generally satisfying results in school achievement levels. A more detailed examination of the information on these three groups of children yielded some surprising results. Although the target group had been accurately matched on the Raven's Matrices with the first control group, there was a very big difference ($p < 0.01$) between these two groups on the Stanford–Binet intelligence test.

| | IQ scores for experimental groups | | |
|---|---|---|---|
| | $T$ | $C_1$ | $C_2$ |
| Mean | 147.100 | 134.343 | 119.200 |
| Standard deviation | 17.413 | 17.133 | 16.094 |
| Number of children | 70 | 70 | 70 |

This considerable discrepancy probably results from a combination of the following effects:

(1)  The Raven's Matrices constitute an entirely visual test, which is as culture-free as possible, whereas the Stanford–Binet has a large element of verbal ability in it. In fact, the target group had received both earlier and more extensive extra tuition than the control groups and came from more verbally conscious homes, judged by the parents' lives and habits and the number of books in the home.

(2)  The Raven's Matrices were given to the children in group conditions, but the Stanford–Binet has to be given in an inter-view-type, one-to-one situation. Results might have been affected by the ease and familiarity with which children in the different groups coped with this 'conversation' with an adult for the latter test.

(3)  There is a 'ceiling' effect in the Raven's Matrices test with highly educated children. This means that the test does not provide a range of measurement among children who are both very bright and culturally fortunate and score in the top 5% of the population on this test. In fact, over three-quarters of the T and $C_1$ group children scored in the top 5% of the possible scores, and over a third of the $C_2$ children. Thus, nearly two-thirds of all the children were in the top 5% of the normal population and needed a finer measure of the effects of their educational background to distinguish

between them. This was largely provided by the Stanford-Binet test.*

Of course, as two tests were used, one for screening and one for individual testing, there would inevitably be differences in their results. But these differences were much bigger than might have been expected. It was for the reasons outlined earlier in this chapter, particularly the greater precision of the Stanford–Binet at the higher levels, that the IQ was used in further investigation as the measure of intellectual ability.

At this point, it was clear that there were now not one, but two differences between the target and first control groups. Firstly, as had been planned, it was only the parents of the target group who had joined the association for gifted children. Secondly, the target children were found to have, on average, a higher IQ than their most closely matched fellow pupils. It looked as though these parents were well aware of their children's very high intelligence and wanted to do something about it. The question now was why they had sought membership of this association. It has been shown that they were generally in a highly favourable position in society and could provide handsomely for their children in every way; yet by their action, they seemed to be trying for something else.

## Home background

The most interesting results of this project were probably those which came from the long interview with the parents. Analysis of the information they provided showed that the parents in the target and two control groups often gave different responses to the questions.

The differences between the parents' answers to the questionnaire, which are outlined below, were all highly significant ($p < 0.01$). This means that the likelihood of the differences turing up by chance were, in most cases, well under 1 in 1000. Since the likelihood of a chance effect was so extremely small, it could be assumed that the differences between the groups were real.

In the parents' descriptions of themselves, there were few big differences between the two control groups. But there were considerable differences between the target and control groups. The variables shown below are only those which showed a marked difference ($p < 0.01$)

* In general, the correlation (relationship) between the two measures is good, varying with the groups of children being tested, e.g. whether they are maladjusted or culturally different ($r$ varies from 0.6 to 0.9). But up among these very able children, the correlation became only moderate ($r = 0.433$) for the standardized scores.

between the target and either of the two control groups. The percentages given are rounded off to the nearest whole number.

| *Mother* | *Experimental groups* | | |
|---|---|---|---|
| | $T$ | $C_1$ | $C_2$ |
| High status occupation | 53 | 33 | 30 |
| Bitter about own education | 14 | 4 | none |
| Reads a lot | 46 | 27 | 16 |
| Reads widely | 31 | 29 | 13 |
| Wide variety of interests | 36 | 21 | 10 |
| Solely responsible for liaison with school | 13 | none | 6 |
| | | (in percentages of 70) | |

The mothers of the sample children were intriguing. Although they had all received a good education, the mothers of the target group had had more university-type experience than the other groups. Yet in spite of (or perhaps because of) this, they showed a distinct and significant element of dissatisfaction with their education. A significant proportion even described themselves as 'bitter'.

These feelings of disappointment about their education seemed even more surprising when related to their work. Over half the target mothers were engaged in professional or top managerial work. By the standards of the general population, where only a tiny percentage of women enjoy such positions, it would seem that they had put their education and abilities to very good use.

The mothers of the target children were clearly a very lively group; they gave the impression of constant activity. The reading of the professional women, such as doctors, was largely confined to vocational literature, as it is with similar men. But they did also find time to read wider material, e.g. biographies, novels and history, while their husbands read fewer books and of narrower range. The mothers' hobbies and activities were very varied. Many of them were involved in non-vocational courses at evening school, several polished pebbles and made jewellery for presents, many were active in traditional women's activities such as sewing and one re-upholstered furniture in her spare time. They were a group of lively and interesting women.

These target mothers also seemed to take a considerable load of responsibility for the family. Their husbands were often away on business so that matters concerning the children's upbringing and education tended to be left to them. It is a well-recognized feature of contemporary professional life that husbands have to become considerably occupied in their careers, leaving the wives to cope with the other things as well as they can. Less pressed husbands may take a greater share of the running of the household, at least in Western society. The target parents seemed to fall very much into the pattern described by the Rapoports in their descriptions of two-career families (Rapoport and Rapoport, 1971; Rapoport *et al.*, 1977). Both parents work hard at their own careers, but it is still the mother who takes the final responsibility for the domestic side of life.

| Father | Experimental groups | | |
|---|---|---|---|
|  | $T$ | $C_1$ | $C_2$ |
| High status occupation | 69 | 60 | 49 |
|  | (in percentages of 70) | | |

No less than 69% of the target fathers were in professional and top managerial positions and the first control group were not far behind at 60%. This may be compared to the general population, in which about 10% of men occupy these positions.

The fathers in the three groups had had very similar educations, so that there was little to choose between them in this respect. On average, 38% had received some form of tertiary education, such as college or university. However, the fathers of the target group were moderately less satisfied with the education they had received than the two control groups – though not as unhappy with it as their wives were with theirs.

Clearly, the target and control-one fathers had been far more successful in their career achievements than the control-two fathers. As it was the mothers of the target group who had achieved considerably more success than either of the control groups, the target parents presented a picture of highly achievement-orientated couples.

However, fathers did not devote their entire lives to their careers; they also had many outside interests, but not as many as their wives. Target fathers had moderately more interests than the control group fathers. So, although they were much more highly achieving, they were also more active in general. Their interests often lay in the more 'masculine' fields, such as cars and sport, but there were plenty of the more general interests, such as bird watching, photography, nature study, music appreciation and genealogy.

| *Both parents* | *Experimental groups* | | |
|---|---|---|---|
| | $T$ | $C_1$ | $C_2$ |
| Parent's fathers had high status occupations | 36 | 24 | 24 |
| Belong to a library | 76 | 69 | 49 |
| Consider music and art very important in education | 28 | 5 | 8 |
| Give specific help with schoolwork | 37 | 16 | 17 |
| Expect child to stay in education till 21 years old | 81 | 60 | 40 |
| Think child is outstanding | 71 | 30 | 21 |
| Unhappy with child's school | 23 | 16 | 8 |
| Very positive educational attitudes | 37 | 23 | 6 |
| Strong pressure on child to achieve | 30 | 13 | 6 |
| | (in percentages of 70) | | |

The fathers of the target group children had clearly improved on their own fathers' career statuses. But the target children's grandfathers were still in a much better position than the control children's grandfathers. So that even a generation ago, there was a difference in social position between the target and control groups. The grandmothers' occupations had also been taken into account, but very little difference emerged between the groups in this respect. Perhaps the social pressures on women a generation ago affected the three groups of grandmothers equally as women, whereas their husbands' careers had the opportunity to be different. The grandmothers' careers, where they existed at all, had largely been confined to the female occupations of secretary, typist, clerk, etc. Most of the grandmothers were full-time housewives, but as many as 13% (on average between the three groups) had held high-status positions such as doctor, teacher, factory manager. Both the grandfathers and grandmothers of these sample children must have been quite influential in the subsequent family life styles looked at in this project, because of their relatively high social status.

In addition to the interests of the mothers and fathers, described separately above, the parents also shared interests and concerns. One of these joint interests showed considerable differences between the groups. Although it was the target group mothers who appeared to be particularly keen on reading, both the parents of the target and the control-one groups had considerably greater membership of a public library. Of course, membership does not necessarily mean use, but the probability is that the mothers of the target children used their library tickets much more than either their husbands or the parents of the other two groups.

The parents of the different groups showed very different attitudes to various aspects of education. The target parents were nearly four times as keen on music and art as being very important parts of their children's education, compared with either of the control groups. Each target child had been matched with the two control children from the same school class, so that the three target children who were at a specialist music school also had 'musical' controls. This specialism could not have affected the results; target parents did have very different aesthetic considerations from the control parents. The figures for attitudes to music and art had been collected separately, but as they were virtually the same for all groups, they are presented here as a combined aesthetic interest.

The parents of the target group gave very much more specific help to their children than the other two groups. This is in contrast to more general, undifferentiated help which all the parents gave about equally. It was very possible that target parents were more able to give specific help because of their own higher level of education, but they were also much more ready and willing to spend time with their children, discussing and explaining problems which had arisen from school work.

This extra help which they gave could have been tied up with their feelings about the school. The target parents were very much less happy with the child's school than the control parents. Again, it must be remembered that all three matched children attended the same school and were in the same class. The parents were, however, less than clear as to why they did not like the schools.

As might have been expected, the parents who had joined the association for gifted children were over twice as likely as other parents to describe their child as outstanding. What is perhaps surprising is that more of them did not do so. Perhaps they were overcome with modesty in the face of the interviewer.

The extent to which the parents saw education as a long-term process is reflected in the percentages who expected their children to stay on in education until they were at least 21 years old. Target parents were keenest on this, followed by control-one and control-two parents in that order. The parents' hopes for their children's future careers were not as outstandingly different as those for their education, but followed the same pattern.

The last two variables in the list given above were subjective; that is, they were judged by the researcher. Their judgement was made on the information available, but also on the impression obtained from visiting the home. These variables were compared between the two researchers, who originally visited the homes together to check the reliability of their ratings. Had there been any discrepancy between these, the variables in question would have been dropped from the research. Not only was there complete agreement between researchers on these matters, but the two variables fell exactly into the pattern which finally emerged of differences between the three groups. For these reasons, they were considered to be entirely valid and acceptable measures.

Target parents did provide a much more positive educational atmosphere in their homes than the control parents, but they also put considerable pressure on the child to achieve success in school. This pressure was almost palpable in some homes and the researchers were glad to have the freedom to leave them. The children could not, of course. This pressure was judged by such remarks as the following:

'We make sure that he sees all the theatre productions and visits the museum and art galleries at least once a month.' (There was no indication of possible pleasure in these activities).

'John's a brilliant boy and of course one of us sits with him every night while he does his homework. Oh yes, (in response to questioning) we have a daughter too, but she's such a silly girl.'

'We don't allow them to watch television at all; they should be doing other things. But sometimes they see it at their friends'.' (Said without a glimmer of humour).

'Of course, he will go to boarding school when he's seven. I can't bear the thought of it, but he has to have the extra tuition which he will get there, to get on in the world. The local school is just ordinary.'

'He doesn't need friends. They only pull him down.'

| The home | Experimental groups | | |
|---|---|---|---|
| | T | $C_2$ | $C_1$ |
| Four or more musical instruments | 31 | 23 | 13 |
| Mostly serious music is played | 41 | 16 | 7 |
| Over 50 books in the home | 63 | 50 | 31 |
| | | | (in percentages of 70) |

These descriptive variables listed above were the only ones which distinguished any of the target group's homes from those of any other group. There were no big differences in the standard of housing between the groups. About 20% of the entire sample lived in superior accommodation, in very pleasant residential areas. Target families were moderately more concerned with the decoration of their homes and hung more pictures up than the control families.

The most significant difference between the homes was due to the families' activities of listening to and practising music. The musically orientated families sometimes had over a dozen instruments in the house. One even had two pianos, one upstairs and one downstairs; they were for the two daughters, in case they were inspired to play at the same time. Musical homes had a great amount of musical equipment; hifi speakers, turntables and tape decks often dominated the living room. The musical families seemed to spend a high proportion of their money on musical activities, which of course included attending and playing in concerts.

Of course, parents' descriptions of their children must always be subjective to some extent. But as I have indicated earlier all measurement, no matter how scientific, has a subjective, personal element in it. To describe a toddler's walking as early or late is a matter of judgement. Walking can be judged as being anything from the first step, but sometimes a child will take two steps and not repeat them again for as much as a month. Many of the aims of this investigation were concerned with parents' ideas and attitudes; their memories and the judgements made from them are considered to be part of the whole package. Parents' judgements of when a child did what, or how they were assessed as behaving, were accepted entirely at face value within the context of this research.

There could be no doubt, however, as to whether each child was a first-born or only child. The target children fell twice as often into this category, but it was surprising that more of these highly intelligent and achieving children did not do so. The literature on gifted children often points out the high prevalence of first-born and only children among them. There would presumably be twice as much of the parental anxiety and the usual first-born problems among the target group than the controls, but the proportion among the total sample was not high.

Significantly more target parents than controls said that their children were noticed as being particularly alert at birth. This is a feature which has also been pointed out in the literature, notably Gesell *et al.* (1965).

The target children were observed as walking and talking earlier than the control groups. Walking was measured by the child's ability to go alone from one side of a room to the other. Talking was measured by the child's ability to produce a short sentence.

The target families were particularly notable in their devotion to 'serious' music. All musical tastes were considered as equal in the research, but the results reflected a distinct musical way of life.

The figure of 50 books was not arbitrary as a cut-off measure for the number of books in a home. There were homes without a single book, and homes where there were more than a thousand. As the research progressed, this figure of 50 seemed to be a reasonable rating, which would distinguish between different kinds of homes; it did indeed prove to be so. There were clear differences between the three groups as to the number of books they possessed. The figures shown above tied up very well with the parents' and children's reading habits. Target families, followed by control-one families, followed by control-two families, were relatively more interested in the world of literature. In fact, music and reading seemed to be the target families' main leisure pursuits, to a much greater extent than either of the control groups.

## The children

The information which has been presented above has all been concerned with the parents' descriptions of themselves and their homes. What follows is the parents' descriptions of their children.

The target children were found to be first-born or only children about twice as often compared with their controls. The prevalence of these children among the gifted and high achievers has been noted before and this finding seemed to provide further supportive evidence for it. Parents of the target children were quite clear as to their child's alertness at birth, though the mother sometimes insisted that this was not her own perception, but that of the nurses or other mothers where the baby was delivered and the baby concerned would be described as 'bright' or 'clever'. Two-thirds of the target parents described their children in this way, though only half of the control-one parents did so. In contrast not one of the control-two parents, who did have some gifted children among their families, described their children as particularly alert at birth. As this description is necessarily subjective, it is possible that expectation, hope or high parental pride in this high proportion of first-born or only children played a part in the description of their first moments of independent life. Further investigation was necessary to find out whether the described alertness at birth is in any way related to giftedness in children.

| The children: development | Experimental groups | | |
| --- | --- | --- | --- |
| | $T$ | $C_1$ | $C_2$ |
| First-born or only child | 13 | 6 | 7 |
| Noticably more alert at birth | 67 | 50 | none |
| Walked early | 67 | 47 | 54 |
| Talked early | 57 | 24 | 16 |
| Read early | 34 | 44 | 29 |
| | | | (in percentages of 70) |

This described neonatal alertness of the target children seemed to be justified by the speed at which they passed their developmental milestones. The criterion for walking was the ability of the baby to cross independently from one side of a room to another. The developmental norms described by Gesell (1950) were used to define whether a child was early, normal or late in his milestones. The target children were described as walking and talking earlier than the control children. For both talking and reading the criterion used was the ability to construct or read a whole sentence.

After all this consistent talent shown by target toddlers, it was very surprising to discover that their parents did not describe them as reading earlier than the control-one group. After all, they did seem to have a good deal more educational investment, and early reading is very often taken as a sure sign of giftedness in itself. The control-one children could not have been described in any way as *more* gifted than the target group and yet they had a significantly earlier age of reading. Even more intriguing was the fact that target parents reported that 1% of their children read at under three years of age, but 6% of the control-one children and 4% of the control-two children were said to have managed it.

| The children: behaviour (parents' descriptions) | Experimental groups | | |
|---|---|---|---|
| | $T$ | $C_1$ | $C_2$ |
| Very 'difficult' | 22 | 3 | 7 |
| Particularly sensitive | 44 | 20 | 15 |
| Very emotional | 19 | 4 | 2 |
| Difficulty with sleep | 50 | 17 | 12 |
| Sleeps little | 6 | 1 | 1 |
| Very independent | 49 | 27 | 13 |
| Feels 'different' | 51 | 3 | 3 |
| No friends | 7 | 1 | 1 |
| Friends older | 36 | 9 | 14 |
| Extraordinary memory | 40 | 19 | 6 |
| Excellent school progress | 43 | 40 | 29 |
| Prefers educational-type TV | 11 | 7 | 4 |
| Wide reading range | 61 | 43 | 33 |
| | (in percentages of 70) | | |

It became quite clear that there were considerable differences in the behaviour of the T group children, as described by their parents, when compared with that of their classmates. The list of child behaviours which emerged was not unlike the lists of behaviours which are supposed to distinguish gifted children.

Over three times as many target as control parents found their children 'very difficult' in general. The answers to this question were often accompanied by parental signs of distress, indicating that 'difficult' was sometimes a euphemism for 'impossible'. Several parents said this difficulty with the child was why they had sought outside help and had therefore chosen the association for gifted children, as it seemed best suited to their needs. Nearly five times as many target parents as controls described their children as very emotional and twice as many described them as particularly sensitive.

The question of sleep was of particular interest since it is the behaviour most often described as distinguishing the gifted from the non-gifted; gifted children are said to need less sleep than others. In this sample, the target parents certainly saw their children as sleeping little. Nearly three times as many target as control children were said to have difficulty with sleep and six times as many were said to sleep significantly less.

Sleep is, of course, a relative matter. When parents belong to a culture in which they feel that six-year-olds should be in bed and asleep by six o'clock, then they will attempt to follow this idea. But if the child does not sleep then the parents can choose to believe there is either something wrong with their idea – or with the child. It may be that the children who sleep 'little' and with difficulty are being put to bed too early for their needs. Quite a number of parents said they were worried about the child's sleeping habits because he was not getting enough sleep and so would do less well at school than he should.

The target children were described as very independent, nearly twice as often as the first control group, but nearly four times as often as the second control group. It may be that the description of 'very independent' is somehow tied up with the description 'very difficult'. I suspect that one may even be substituted for the other, since the same signs and distressed looks prefaced the description of 'independent'. Some parents left their independent children to get on with their own pursuits, but some tried to curb their independence and bring the child back into the conventional fold. I had the impression that this latter approach itself produced more of the difficult behaviour.

It was particularly remarkable that the parents of the target group said their children felt 'different' seventeen times as often as parents of the control group. They could possibly have felt different because of their high intelligence, but then the target and control groups had been exactly matched on the Raven's scale, so that a difference of seventeen times would have been quite out of proportion, even using the Stanford–Binet scores. It was far more likely that the considerable differences in their families and in their own behaviour made the children feel different. They did have a long list of problematic behaviour and added to that was the fact that this was the parents' description. This was not the child's description of himself – it was how his parents thought he felt. Maybe they thought that was how he *should* feel; more investigation was needed.

Target children had very many fewer friends than the control children; 7% had no friends at all, compared with 1% in each of the control groups. Parents often said it was because nobody suitable lived nearby and school was far away. But again, the three children of the triad lived in the same area and went to the same school. They lived in the same kind of house and none of them was physically unattractive. This paucity of friends in the target group could not have been entirely due to these fortuitous reasons that the parents gave for it. In fact, the target children were not really very easy to be friends with and their parents often occupied them after school with scholastic work or visits to worthwhile places, while their peers played outside. The effect of this could hardly have been good for the children, since part of their process of growing up with friends was considerably impaired.

The friends that the target children did have were described, more often than the friends of the control children, as being older rather than the same age or younger. The parents often approved of these friendships, explaining that 'Anne finds it difficult to talk to children of her own age because of her high ability'. One mother said that without his older friends, her son would be 'lost', as there were only children of his own age to talk to otherwise. In spite of this preference for older friends, only two children of the target sample had been pushed up a year at school. One of the control children had also been 'upped' a year. Had more of the target children mixed with older children at school, their older friendships would have been understandable. As it was, either they were at a loss among their own age-group at school, or there were other reasons for having older friends at home, such as rising to parental expectations.

Although so many of the target parents expressed dissatisfaction with their child's school, a high proportion of them said their children were making excellent progress there. The control-two group parents, who had showed the least worry about the school, saw their children as making the least progress. The parents of the target children, however, seemed to want someting more from the school. There was also a small proportion, about 6%, equally across all the groups, who were not doing well. The children in all three groups ranged from gifted to average ability.

The children's leisure habits, as described by their parents, were distinct in two particular ways. The target children were described as watching more educational-type television, such as documentaries, and as having a preference for BBC2 (the most intellectual channel) or topics of current interest. General entertainment came very low on their lists. They were also said to read widely and often in preference to television. Some parents said their children 'never' watched it, adding that 'it is such a waste of time; there are much better things to do'. Other children were officially restricted by their parents from watching television, to varying extents.

## The children's descriptions of themselves

The questionnaire given to the children was not long. With hindsight, it was concluded that it should have been longer and the questions would then have mirrored more accurately those given to the parents. However, the information the children did give proved to be very interesting, particularly in relation to the parents' descriptions of the children, outlined above.

While the three groups' parents had described their children, in varying proportions, as reading widely, the children were quite explicit about what they actually preferred reading. Only 1% of the target children preferred to read informative material and none of the others did. Of the three groups, 99% of target children, 97% of control-one children and 97% of control-two children preferred comics to all else.

When asked how they felt about the school they attended, almost all the children responded very positively. Of the target children, 80% were very happy, while 94% of control-one and 84% of control-two children were also very happy. The others had reservations, but none claimed actually to be unhappy at school. Thus, apart from the target parents' feelings about the child's school (23% did not care for it), there was otherwise overwhelming support for the schools.

The differences between the three groups of children, which were all significant at 1% ($p < 0.01$), are listed below.

The control-one children played significantly more sport than the target children. The amount of sport played, as described by the children, was outside the school curriculum. But on the basis of the figures given above, it looks as though the control-one children were out playing football while the target children were indoors practising their musical instruments. As the target children also engaged in more supervised scholastic work, they were probably doing that too.

| The children: self descriptions | Experimental groups | | |
|---|---|---|---|
| | T | $C_1$ | $C_2$ |
| Play competitive sports | 28 | 51 | 37 |
| Play musical instrument(s) | 46 | 29 | 19 |
| Children who suggested more than 1 improvement in teaching | 39 | 96 | 17 |
| Can see life through another's eyes | 19 | 6 | 11 |
| Can pay attention to more than one thing at once | 56 | 21 | 17 |
| | | (in percentages of 70) | |

The children were asked a number of questions about their school life, in particular how they would improve it. The control children gave over twice as many suggestions as the target children. It could be interpreted that the target children had more respect for the school system as it stood and that the control-one children felt freer to make suggestions for change. Target children did not, even in this tangential way, feel as unhappy about their schools as their parents did.

Questions about the children's sensitivity did confirm the parents' opinions that the target children were very sensitive. They were far more able to empathise with other people than the other two groups. But they were not more aware than the others as to how other people might see them. They certainly did not feel liked or disliked by others because of their 'gifts'. They knew how their parents felt about them because they were members of the association for gifted children, but seemed to deny that they were in any way different from the other children in their school class.

More than twice as often as the other two groups the target children said they were able to pay attention to more than one thing at once. Could this, along with their heightened sensitivity to other people, be a sign of the gifted children among them? Fifty-six per cent of them said they could do this, compared with an average 19% of the control groups. Further investigation would no doubt shed some light on this.

## The teachers

The children's own class teachers were asked about their charges' behaviour in class. This was done with the Bristol Social Adjustment Guides (Stott, 1976) which was described in detail earlier (p. 138). It has pre-rated statements, which the teacher has to underline, and spaces to put down spontaneous remarks. The teachers were most often not aware as to which of the children that they were asked to comment on were 'gifted'. Parents did not always tell the teachers about their membership of the association and sometimes asked the researcher not to let the cat out of the bag. It was not considered to be ethical research to have told the teachers of the parents' actions, if they did not want this. In the circumstances, it was quite impossible to be sure of the teachers' opinions as to who was and who was not considered to be gifted; accordingly, that control had to be dropped. The teachers were not asked any other questions beyond what was in the Guides.

There was not one single significant difference between the control groups over the complete range of scores made by the teachers for the children on this measure, on any of the 27 variables. All the variables listed below showed significant differences at 1% ($p < 0.01$) between the target and control groups only, on scores of one or more.

| Children's social adjustment in school | Experimental groups | | |
|---|---|---|---|
| | T | $C_1$ | $C_2$ |
| Under-reaction | | | |
| Withdrawal | 23 | 10 | 10 |
| Non-specific under-reaction | 37 | 24 | 21 |
| Over-reaction | | | |
| Inconsequence | 50 | 26 | 34 |
| Hostility | 39 | 17 | 13 |
| Peer maladaptiveness | 29 | 14 | 9 |
| Total over-reaction | 63 | 54 | 30 |
| | (Scores of $> 1$, in percentages of 70) | | |

These figures represent the scores of each teacher's opinions on the three experimental group members in her class. The percentages overlap considerably because many of the children were assigned to several behavioural categories. One child could, for instance, be hostile and peer-maladaptive, with occasional withdrawal. Any one child would not be expected to show all the signs indicated by the teacher all the time, or all at once. Looking at any class of children, some of them would be more under-reactive than the main body of children, while some would be more over-reactive. These experimental groups of children were subject to the same variation.

In comparison with the control children, the target children were less under-reactive than over-reactive. Some of them showed signs of withdrawal, but their under-reaction was usually less specific. In this respect, they would be less than fully participating members of the school class.

Their high tendency to over-reaction would, however, make the target children very noticeable members of the class. That 50% of them showed signs of inconsequence means that they would act without thinking of the consequence first. This is the sort of behaviour which Stott (1976) believes leads to accident proneness. The children would be inclined to act without thinking first, which would undoubtedly irritate the teachers. Such a child tends to learn by trial and error and to become frustrated and discouraged more easily than other children. Mischief may be a way of avoiding tasks, but it is also antisocial and can be hostile. The target children were much more hostile than their controls (over twice as often) which would make them more difficult for the teacher to cope with. This high level of inconsequence and hostility is a considerable handicap to making good relationships. The teachers were in entire agreement with the parents that the target children were poor at making friends. Twice as many of them as the controls were described as peer-maladaptive.

The total over-reaction score of the T group was by far the highest and there were significant differences between each of the three experimental groups. Nearly two-thirds of the target group were described as over-reactive, over a half of the control-one group and less than a third of the control-two group. Thus, there seemed to be some factor operating effectively across the three groups. The Guides do allow for further investigation into the signs of over-reaction and they are presented below. Only the differences which are significant at 1% are given.

It must perhaps be explained that the percentages of children in the more detailed investigation do not add up to those in the broader categories. There was again overlap across the scores. Thus, although 50% of the target children showed inconsequential behaviour, some of them showed it in both the aspects of hyperactivity and showing off, but some of them would show it in only one of the detailed categories. The 50% of children were not split equally into the two detailed categories, nor did all the 50% fulfil both the categories. In addition, there were some children in categories of the adjustment guides which are not listed above because there were no significant differences between the groups.

| Children's over-reaction | Experimental groups | | |
|---|---|---|---|
| | $T$ | $C_1$ | $C_2$ |
| Inconsequence | | | |
| Hyperactivity | 36 | 9 | 11 |
| Showing off | 33 | 9 | 17 |
| Hostility | | | |
| Moody/sullen | 31 | 11 | 10 |
| Provocative | 10 | 1 | 3 |
| Aggressive | 23 | 7 | 3 |
| Peer maladaptiveness | | | |
| Aggressive | 9 | 4 | 0 |
| | (scores of $> 1$ in percentages of 70) | | |

One-third of the target group was seen by their teachers as being not just lively, but actually hyperactive. One-third was also seen as showing off.

The hostility of the target group was then looked at in more detail. As a group, they showed over twice as much distressing or distressed signs of general hostility than the control groups. Moody/sullenness affected almost a third of them, added to which their high level of aggressiveness and downright provocativeness cannot have made them endearing.

The target group's lack of friends appeared to be due to the underlying hostility in many of them. The teacher's descriptions of all the children's friendships were overall in entire agreement with those of the parents. This gave much more validity to the probability that it was the children's aggression which was responsible for their lack of friends.

These comparisons provide a highly dramatic picture of the target and control children's behaviour in school. As pupils, the target children would be expected to have been very much less attractive to their teachers, as well as to their classmates, than the control children. They could be easily distinguished from the rest of the class by their difficult behaviour. Parents and teachers were in very close agreement as to the characteristic quality of difficulty shown by these children, although the children themselves did not feel themselves to be different from other children

## Additional information

There was more information to be picked from the bones of the major measuring instruments which added to the growing evidence of the differences between the three groups. This information had not been specifically requested and pre-rated; it was gleaned from the parent's and teacher's responses. The evidence from all the parents did not provide information on all the points concerned, but the evidence from the teachers was uniform, thanks to the presentation of the Adjustment Guides which they filled in.

The health of the children was particularly noteworthy.

| Children's physical health | Experimental groups | | | | | |
|---|---|---|---|---|---|---|
| | $T$ | | $C_1$ | | $C_2$ | |
| | Teachers | Parents | Teachers | Parents | Teachers | Parents |
| Stomach complaints | 4 | 3 | 4 | 1 | 3 | 1 |
| Respiratory/nervous complaints | 11 | 24 | 3 | 24 | 6 | 16 |
| Speech problems | 11 | 1 | 9 | 0 | 11 | 4 |
| Poor eyesight | 13 | 0 | 6 | 3 | 6 | 0 |
| Poor coordination | 9 | 16 | 1 | 3 | 1 | 3 |
| Totals | 48 | 44 | 31 | 30 | 30 | 24 |
| Average percentage reported | 46 | | 27 | | 27 | |
| | | | (in percentages of 70) | | | |

The teachers tended to describe more problems than the parents. This could have been due to differences in the collecting procedure or to reticence or preconceptions on the part of the parents. For example, 13% of target children were described as having poor eyesight by their teachers, while only 1% of parents reported this. Also, many more speech problems were reported by the teachers than by the parents for all groups. These qualifications applied equally, of course, to the three groups. Although it may not be precisely accurate, the table above provides an acceptably correct picture of the reported physical health of the three experimental groups. It shows that there are over one and a half times as many physical problems amongst the target group as amongst the control groups. The target group seemed to be particularly prone to poor coordination and had rather more problems with respiratory troubles than the other two groups. This list of physical complaints (apart from poor eyesight) is indicative of anxiety in children.

It is often found in research that children of very high social status and ability are more attractive to their teachers than their classmates. However the teachers in this study did not differentiate between the children in these respects.

| *Children's attractiveness* | *Experimental groups* | | |
|---|---|---|---|
| | $T$ | $C_1$ | $C_2$ |
| Attractive | 41 | 49 | 49 |
| Not so attractive | 10 | 4 | 11 |
| | (in percentages of 70) | | |

The teachers could not be accused of singling out the children they liked least to complain of in the questionnaire.

Investigation of the children's sleep patterns added weight to the picture of general disturbance among the target children.

| *Children's sleep patterns* | *Experimental groups* | | |
|---|---|---|---|
| | $T$ | $C_1$ | $C_2$ |
| Disturbed sleep | 34 | 10 | 11 |
| Symptoms resulting in disturbed sleep | 20 | 4 | 6 |
| | (in percentages of 70) | | |

The symptoms which resulted in disturbed sleep, given by the parents, included head battering, bed-wetting, forgetting hypnotics, sleep walking, fear of the dark and nightmares. Again, the target children had at least three times as many of these as the control children.

Information from the parent's interview about the family backgrounds of the groups could only be asked for and accepted at face value. Parents in the North-West of England are not always happy about disclosing old family skeletons. Consequently the figures offered below are probably an under-estimate, but of course this would apply equally to all three groups.

| Unusual home backgrounds | Experimental groups | | |
|---|---|---|---|
| | T | $C_1$ | $C_2$ |
| Remarriage | 9 | 6 | 1 |
| One-parent family | 7 | 0 | 1 |
| Adopted child | 1 | 3 | 3 |
| Siblings over 7 years older | 4 | 4 | 5 |
| | | (percentage of 70) | |

Here again, the target group children were found to have about twice as many instances of unusual family backgrounds as either of the control groups. The children of one-parent families were seven times as prevalent in the target group. Such parents, being on their own, would be expected to seek outside help more often than those of stable marriages.

Looking more closely at parents' occupations showed that a very high proportion of the sample were teachers. This included teachers of all sorts, from university professors to nursery school staff.

| Parents who are teachers | Experimental groups | | |
|---|---|---|---|
| | T | $C_1$ | $C_2$ |
| Only mother teaches | 14 | 19 | 7 |
| Only father teaches | 3 | 3 | 4 |
| Both parents teach | 13 | 3 | 6 |
| | | (percentage of 70) | |

*165*

The differences between the groups were not quite as great here as in other aspects of the investigation, but still the target group parents were somewhat more likely to be teachers than either of the control groups. The biggest difference was when both parents were practising teachers, when the target children had over twice the number of teaching parents than either of the control groups. This would seem to have contributed positively to their decision to join the association. There is the probability that teachers, being continually concerned with education, have educational achievement more in mind than other people. This, in combination with the belief that their own child was gifted, would predispose them to join an organization which was concerned with promoting educational facilities for gifted children. In addition, a high proportion of their children's schools were in the private sector (39%), which also indicated that teachers were more likely to choose private schools than other people. In all, 71.43% of the total sample children had at least one parent who was a teacher of some sort.

The target parents had been asked quite specifically why they had joined the National Association for Gifted Children. Their answers were coded as follows:

*Main reasons for joining NAGC* (in percentages of 70)

| Problems | | Other reasons | |
|---|---|---|---|
| At home | 6 | Activities provided | 11 |
| At school | 30 | Curiosity | 6 |
| Insurance against | 13 | My child is 'different' | 33 |
| | | Don't know | 1 |

On the basis of the above coding of the answers, it appears that parents joined equally for problems or for other reasons. But it seems probable that parents who joined because their child was 'different' were concerned with the problems brought about by that difference. This category of reason for joining could equally well be brought under the *Problem* column. The percentage of parents who would have joined for possible problems would then be 82%. The parents who joined as an insurance against future problems explained that although they had no

166

problems at present, they knew that they were likely to have them. Most of them offered the list of behaviour disturbances which are often published as an indication of giftedness in children. They had read about them and were expecting them to befall the child they believed to be gifted. This was a small but clear example of the possible harm which comes about from the spreading of such unfounded opinion.

## Summary of the experimental groups

As a whole, the sample proved to be of high social status. But evidence which came from the comparisons between the target and control groups showed that the target group was very different from the control groups. These differences were apparent on most of the major aspects of the children's home backgrounds and of their behaviour at home and at school. The sources of information from which these comparisons were made were the parents, the children and the class teachers.

Responses to the interview with parents distinguished between the parents of the target and control groups. Although the mothers of the three groups had received similar educations, some of the target mothers were bitter and others were very dissatisfied with theirs, and the target fathers were moderately dissatisfied. Target mothers had far higher status occupations than control mothers; they were also very lively. More of them were solely responsible for school matters than control mothers. Fathers of the target group also had a higher occupational status than the control group, but were not significantly distinguished in any other way.

Both parents of the target group were interested in the arts and reading. They gave considerable educational support to their children, but were not always happy with their children's schools. They were very positive in their attitudes to the prosperity of their children's education, but also put very much stronger pressure on their children to achieve than either of the control groups. The target parents themselves seemed to have achieved successfully in their own fields.

The homes of the target group were more plentifully supplied with books and musical instruments. The target children also had more music lessons than the control children. The target families listened to more serious music than the control families.

The target children were described by their parents as being more alert at birth than the control children were. Their milestones of walking and talking were earlier, but they read later than the control-one children. More of the target children were first-born or only children.

The target parents said that their children were difficult to bring up They described them as particularly sensitive, very emotional, disturbed sleepers who sleep little, and of independent natures many times more frequently than either of the control group parents in their children's descriptions. Parents were clear that their children felt 'different', which was not surprising in view of their behaviour, but the children did not describe themselves as feeling different.

Although they did not always care for their children's school, target parents approved of their progress in it. The target children were said to read widely, to prefer good quality television, but to have a paucity of friends.

The children's own description of themselves was more modest. Most of the sample said they liked to watch sport on television and did not read very much. They all loved comics. The control-one children seemed to be more involved with school in that they made considerably more suggestions about improvements for teaching than the other two children in the same class. They also played more competitive sport. The target children described themselves as sensitive, as being able to empathise with others and able to divide their attention into more than one involvement.

The children's teachers distinguished very specifically and significantly between the three groups. The target children were seen as showing much more troubled behaviour in the classroom than the other two groups. Some of them (23%) were under-reactive, but half (50%) were seen as over-reactive. There was a lot of hostility and aggressiveness in the over-reactive children; they were inconsequential in their thinking and had difficulty in making friends.

Material gleaned from the written, unrated comments in the interviews threw more light on the situation. The target children had over one and a half times as many physical complaints as the control children. They not only slept less well, but had more symptoms of disturbance during the night. The target families were less conventional in their make-up than the control families, such as having more changes in parenting. Teachers featured highly in the occupations of target parents. When asked why they had joined an association for gifted children, the reasons given were mostly because of problems or possible problems.

The target children seemed to be less well adjusted to life than other similarly able children, or their schoolmates. Parents said that they found these children difficult to live with and, in view of their described behaviour and generally very high ability, were fortunate to have an appropriate helping organization to turn to.

# THE IQ GROUPS

The extreme differences between the target and control groups, described above in this chapter, had not been expected at the beginning of the research. However, in both home background and behaviour, the target children were found to be very different from the control children. The adults who were involved with them, i.e. parents and teachers, were in close agreement about the distinctly more difficult behaviour of the target children.

There were three reasons which either singly or in combination could have been responsible for the target children's different behaviour. Firstly, they did have a higher Stanford–Binet IQ score (though not a higher Raven's score) and secondly, their family backgrounds were psychologically different; the third possible reason was that there could have been inherent differences in the children themselves.

The argument that the IQ differences had caused the differences in behaviour was convincing at face value. There was, after all, a significantly higher average IQ among the target group children than among either of the control groups. Most children of such high intelligence are described in the literature as being isolated and unhappy in a normal world. There are many experts who would say that these results were only to be expected; gifted children are by definition abnormal and the target children were very often gifted. It would follow that they would of course be 'different' and, being so, would find life more of a problem than normal children. Consequent difficulties in behaviour would be normal for gifted children.

But having seen both the parents and the children of all three groups and having known them in their own homes, it seemed to me very doubtful that their giftedness alone could be responsible for the children's behaviour. This was for two reasons.

Firstly, the target and control-one children had been accurately matched on the Raven's matrices raw score. This is a test of intellectual ability and does provide an excellent basis for matching children in that respect for research purposes. Using the raw score for matching individual children provides a precise measure of non-verbal ability. There were children of extremely high ability in both these matched groups, but little sign of unhappiness in the control-one group. Secondly, the parents of these two groups of children seemed to be different in their attitudes and ways of life. From general knowledge of child development, it was assumed that these parental differences must have had some effect on their children.

Virtually no evidence emerged from the research as to any inherent differences between the three experimental groups of children. Doubtless their detailed medical histories would have provided some relevant information, though what is inborn and what is learned must very often be a matter of inference. In this research, the significant evidence came in relation to the children in their social environments. The next stage of the investigation was designed to separate the effects of high IQ by itself from high IQ along with other possible influences.

If there were behaviour differences in children caused by high IQ alone, then they should have been observable, since IQ varied from the children of average ability to those who were intellectually gifted. It was also possible to examine whether there was any qualitative distinction between bright and very gifted children. Above all, the quest was for a point along the available IQ range which could possibly be used in the identification of gifted children. If it became clear, for example, that behaviour and outlook changed significantly between, say IQ 140 and IQ 150, then it would be justifiable to make a more precise definition of intellectual giftedness than had been available so far.

In order to investigate the possibility of behavioural change varying with IQ, the information which had been collected about the children was ordered according to their measured IQ, from the lowest to the highest scores. For convenience of measurement, the children were compared in steps of ten IQ points from IQ 100 or less to IQ 170, which was the upper limit of the test. The whole sample appeared in IQ terms in the table opposite.

The differences in IQ between the three original groups can now be seen more clearly. Some of the children who were presented by their parents as gifted had only moderate IQs. Although this is not the only measure of giftedness, such relatively low scores were surprising. Each of these ten steps was compared with every other step on all the variables.

It is often asked whether children who are intellectually precocious become less so as they grow older. By far the best way to judge this is to re-measure such children over the years. However, as there was a selection of children in this sample aged from five to thirteen years, a cross-section of their intelligence levels could have been informative. There was, in fact, no change of IQ among the children of different ages.

The Stanford–Binet test scores are adjusted for age and even this unusual sample was accommodated within its statistical structure.

The sample was examined to see whether IQ and the sex of the child were related. However, there was no significant difference between the boys' and the girls' IQs.

The mother's age at the birth of the child is known to be a considerable factor in the likelihood of a child being born mentally impaired. Therefore, there has been speculation as to whether gifted children are more likely to be born to older mothers. In fact, no relationship was found between the mother's age at the birth and the child's I.Q. Nor had there been any relationship between the mothers' ages in any of the three experimental groups.

However, there were differences in both behaviour and life-styles between children among the IQ range. The greater the disparity of IQ between the children, the greater their life differences. This can be seen in the graph overleaf, which compares the number of differences between the groups on all the variables, with the range of IQ in 10-point steps.

| IQ range | Experimental groups | | | Totals |
|----------|-----|-----|-----|--------|
| | $T$ | $C_1$ | $C_2$ | |
| 100 or less | — | 1 | 7 | 8 |
| 101 – 110 | — | 2 | 15 | 17 |
| 111 – 120 | 5 | 14 | 21 | 40 |
| 121 – 130 | 8 | 13 | 16 | 37 |
| 131 – 140 | 10 | 14 | 2 | 26 |
| 141 – 150 | 14 | 13 | 6 | 33 |
| 151 – 160 | 15 | 8 | 3 | 26 |
| 161 – 170 | 18 | 5 | — | 23 |
| Totals | 70 | 70 | 70 | 210 |
| | (Actual numbers) | | | |

It can be seen from the graph that the greatest number of differences between the IQ steps occurred between the lowest and the highest IQs. Had a lower range of IQ been included than the sample offered, the curve of the graph would probably have been balanced equally on both sides. This uniformity of behaviour differences along with IQ differences provides evidence of the validity and suitability of the measurements in this research.

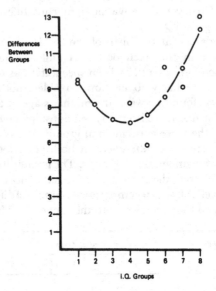

*Behaviour differences related to steps of 10 IQ points*

The most important finding from this overall look at the sample in respect of IQ was that IQ and behaviour are related in terms of the whole environment. But the relationship does not change suddenly between IQ points or groups of points. It continues smoothly from average to high intelligence. The search for an area of intelligence in which it would be possible to define a gifted child was not fulfilled here; no acceptable cut-off point was found in the terms of this enquiry.

## The high and moderate intelligence groups

A more precise investigation was needed of the differences which had been found in both the children and their backgrounds, when grouped according to levels of intelligence quotient. To do this, all the children of the sample were taken out of their original categories of target and control groups. They were then re-sorted on the basis of their measured

172

Stanford–Binet IQs into two new groups. A working figure of IQ 141 was taken as being high, so that children who scored 141 or more were placed in the High IQ group, ranging from 141 to 170. Children who scored below this were placed in the Moderate IQ group, ranging from 140 to 97. The following two groups emerged.

| *IQ scores* | *IQ groups* | |
|---|---|---|
| | *High* | *Moderate* |
| Mean | 155.012 | 119.797 |
| Standard deviation | 9.903 | 11.589 |
| Number of children | 82 | 128 |

The original three experimental groups had each contained 70 children. But the proportions of children in the new groups were changed; the Moderate IQ group now had 128 children, one and a half times as many children as the High IQ group, which contained 82 children. The original experimental groups, re-sorted into the intelligence groups, are shown below in percentages of their new groups.

| *Experimental groups* | *IQ groups* | |
|---|---|---|
| | *High* | *Moderate* |
| Target | 57.32 | 17.97 |
| Control-one | 31.70 | 34.38 |
| Control-two | 10.98 | 47.66 |

(in percentages of 82 and 128)

The original target children formed well over half the new High IQ group, whereas the control-one group formed just under a third and the control-two group a tenth. It would be expected that those variables which had distinguished the target group from its controls would be likely to reappear in this comparison because of the large proportion of target children in the High IQ group. Where they did not appear, it was considered that the new differences between the High and Moderate IQ groups were true differences between these groups of children and families. The new differences would – in a sense – have overridden the influence of the large proportion of target children in the High IQ group and would be due to the essential criterion of measured IQ.

Further statistical comparisons were made between the High and Moderate IQ groups with reference to all the data from the parents, schools and children. The High IQ group, containing 82 children with an average IQ of 155, provided an unusually good sample of children who would be included, by any definition, among the gifted.

## Home background

Many significant differences were found in the comparison of the High and Moderate IQ groups. The presentation of comparisons is arranged in the same way as that between the target and control groups. The variables recorded here are only those which showed a marked difference ($p < 0.01$) between the High and Moderate IQ groups. The percentages given are rounded off to the nearest whole number.

| *Mother* | *IQ groups* | |
|---|---|---|
| | *High* | *Moderate* |
| High status occupation | 57 | 27 |
| High level of education | 50 | 22 |
| Reads a lot | 43 | 21 |
| Reads widely | 35 | 17 |
| Wide variety of interests | 34 | 13 |
| | (In percentages of 82 and 128) | |

The mothers of the High IQ group had a very high level of education and occupation, both in comparison to the Moderate IQ mothers and to the population in general. Compared to the mothers of Moderate IQ children, they were avid and wide readers and had considerably more general interests. But unlike the mothers of the target group, when compared with their controls, this comparison did not show the mothers of the High IQ group as being dissatisfied, much less bitter about their own education. Nor were these mothers found to be solely responsible for the relationship with the child's school more often than the Moderate IQ mothers, as the target group mothers had been in comparison with their controls.

The mothers of the high IQ children appeared to be a quite exceptional group themselves. They were high achievers, who led interesting and varied lives. Their general satisfaction seemed to be founded on a very lively and favourable way of life.

| Father | IQ groups | |
|---|---|---|
| | High | Moderate |
| High status occupation | 78 | 47 |
| High level of education | 50 | 30 |
| Reads a lot | 34 | 16 |
| Read widely | 24 | 15 |
| Wide variety of interests | 37 | 13 |
| | (in percentages of 82 and 128) | |

The fathers of the High IQ group proved to be of a superior social level, their occupations and education being appropriate. In comparison with the Moderate IQ group, their leisure hours were very much more lively and varied. When the target fathers had been compared to the control fathers, the only big differences had been in the fathers' occupations. In this case, the High IQ group fathers showed a much broader and fuller life, when compared to the Moderate IQ group fathers. Like the mothers, they were also very high achievers. The same proportion of High IQ mothers and fathers had received higher education (50%), but the fathers had had considerably more success in their careers. Their leisure interests were of a similar nature and amount to those of the mothers.

The children of the High IQ group had come from a more socially elevated background than the Moderate IQ group, from as long ago as their grandparents' time. Grandfathers especially, but grandmothers too, had been of significantly higher occupational status.

The general cultural level of the High IQ group parents was much higher than that of the Moderate IQ parents. A far greater proportion of them belonged to a library and appeared to make use of it liberally and with enjoyment. They were concerned nearly four times as often as the Moderate IQ group parents that music and art were essential in the broad education of their young.

The High IQ group parents were not only concerned about their children's education, but went to a great deal of trouble to make sure that it was the best that they could provide. The High IQ children did have considerably more help outside school than the Moderate IQ children. Their parents had been assiduous in teaching their children, from the time they were born; they taught them to count and read before they went to school. Once there, the children received more help from their parents, both generally and in specific subjects. They also had extra professional lessons outside school hours; these were mostly music, but also included art and some scholastic tuition.

| Both parents | IQ groups | |
| --- | --- | --- |
| | High | Moderate |
| Parents' parents had high status occupations | 30 | 18 |
| Belong to a library | 84 | 52 |
| Consider music and art important in education | 38 | 10 |
| Give child help – before school | 64 | 56 |
| – specific teaching | 49 | 30 |
| – extra lessons | 60 | 41 |
| Expect child to stay in education till 21 years old | 88 | 13 |
| Think child is outstanding | 56 | 31 |
| Positive educational attitudes | 38 | 12 |
| Pressure on child to achieve | 24 | 11 |
| | (in percentages of 82 and 128) | |

The considerable investment which their parents were putting into the education of these children was undoubtedly purposeful. Nearly seven times as many High IQ as Moderate IQ children were expected to stay in the educational system until they were at least 21 years old. This difference in the level of expectation between these two groups was very much higher than any other comparison between the groups. High IQ group parents, when compared to the parents of the Moderate IQ group, did not consider their child to be outstanding as often as might have been expected, although their positive educational attitudes were.

about three times more pronounced. Also, their pressure on the child to achieve was about double, but, considering the vast amount of educational expertise that was being poured into these children, as well as the parents' great expectations for them, the pressure on the children could have been much more powerful than it actually was. By comparison, the original target parents had exerted three times as much pressure on their children as the combined controls.

| The home | IQ groups | |
|---|---|---|
| | High | Moderate |
| Four or more musical instruments | 35 | 14 |
| Music noticeably important | 38 | 17 |
| Mostly serious music played | 32 | 15 |
| Quality newspapers taken | 38 | 17 |
| Over 50 books in home | 72 | 33 |
| Superior neighbourhood | 82 | 60 |
| | (in percentages of 81 and 128) | |

About a third of all the High IQ group homes were occupied with matters of serious music – both listening and making it. This was about the same proportion as in the target homes, but the difference was that in the High IQ group, music was more noticeably important in their homes. This meant that there were more hifi sets installed, more instruments to be seen, more sheet music in view ready to be played.

The homes of the High IQ group were twice as likely to take serious, good quality, newspapers than the Moderate IQ group. This concern with good quality reading is reflected in the number of books in the home, which the High IQ families had in profusion. The parents' reading habits were further evidence of their concern with the written word.

As would be expected with the superior socio-economic status of the parents, the High IQ families lived in the better neighbourhoods of their towns more often than the Moderate IQ parents. The picture of the High IQ home which emerged was that of a detached house in a pleasant suburb, a book-lined interior and music floating on the air.

## The children

All the information presented in this section has been of the parents' descriptions of themselves and their homes. What follows is the parents' descriptions of their children. Only where there is a 1% difference between the two groups is the variable presented.

| The children: development | IQ groups | |
|---|---|---|
| | *High* | *Moderate* |
| Talked early | 45 | 24 |
| Read early | 67 | 35 |
| | (in percentages of 82 and 128) | |

There were only two distinct differences in the development of the children in the High and Moderate IQ groups that were reported by their parents. The High IQ children were described as having talked very much earlier and having been able to read a short sentence very much earlier. The validity of early reading as a sign of intellectual giftedness was considerably strengthened by this finding. Of the High IQ group, 27% were said to be reading a little by the time they were three years old, but only 5% of the Moderate IQ group were said to be as precocious. This was a remarkable difference. It was interesting that it was the verbal aspects of children's developments which were most prominent in this comparison, but then the results of the children's IQ, used to form the groups, were from a test which has a high verbal component.

Particularly noticeable by its absence in this comparison was the prevalence of first born or only children among the High IQ groups. This variable had, however, been significant at the 1% level when the target children had been compared to their controls. In addition, the target parents had reported that their children were more alert at birth than other babies (67%), which also proved to be very significantly different from the reports of the control parents. There was apparently no difference between the High and Moderate IQ groups in respect of their alertness at birth. Whether children were first born or only was a matter of fact, but whether they were alert at birth is a matter of perception – in this case, by the parents.

The next matter to be investigated was that of the children's behaviour, as described by their parents. Considerable differences between the target children and their controls emerged here. However, only those differences which were significant at 1% ($p < 0.01$) are presented.

| The children: Behaviour (parents' descriptions) | IQ groups | |
|---|---|---|
| | High | Moderate |
| More lively than other children | 33 | 44 |
| Very independent | 38 | 24 |
| Child feels decidedly different | 35 | 9 |
| No friends | 5 | 3 |
| Friends older | 30 | 13 |
| Extraordinary memory | 35 | 13 |
| Can concentrate for many hours | 26 | 10 |
| Excellent school progress | 54 | 27 |
| Poor handwriting | 37 | 18 |
| Wide variety of creative interests | 28 | 16 |
| Reads widely | 63 | 34 |
| High status occupation expected | 28 | 13 |
| | (in percentages of 82 and 128) | |

The list of problematical behaviours, as described by the parents of the target children, which were significantly more plentiful than in the control children, did not show significant differences in this above comparison. But there were other variables which did distinguish most significantly between the High IQ and Moderate IQ group.

It was the Moderate IQ children who were described as livelier. Therefore, assumptions about gifted children being more lively than average children do not appear to hold, at least for this sample. However, the High IQ children were certainly seen as much more independent and were described nearly four times as often as feeling 'different'. Parents obviously empathised with this feeling of their children, though most often the children did not claim it. In this comparison, the children were indeed of gifted ability, when compared to the other children, and consequently could be reasonably expected to feel different.

Although the percentages of children involved were low, there were more High IQ children without friends than Moderate IQ children. However, when the High IQ children did have friends, these were over twice as likely as the Moderate IQ children's friends to be older. Thus, the likelihood of the highly intelligent child having few, but older friends, does seem to be true for these children.

The High IQ group were said to have extraordinary good memories and displayed great feats of concentration about three times as often as the Moderate IQ children. These two features are also frequently mentioned as indicative of intellectual giftedness. It was not surprising that over half the High IQ children were said to be making excellent progress in school. However, over one-third of them were said to have poor handwriting, compared to only a fifth of the Moderate group. This latter is a feature of gifted children often mentioned by teachers, but not yet documented.

The High IQ children were said to have a wide variety of creative interests. They painted, modelled, made collections and went on explorations nearly twice as much as the Moderate IQ children, but read widely in about the same proportion. This activity was paralleled in the two groups in the whole literary outlook of the family. The number of books in the house, the parents' membership of a library and mother's and father's reading habits, all amounted to the fact that there was twice as much going on in the High IQ group families as in the Moderate IQ group families.

As might have been expected, the parents of the High IQ children anticipated a higher status occupation for their children much more frequently than the parents of the Moderate IQ group. This was very much in keeping with the differences between the two groups, in the parents' and grandparents' occupations, which varied between one and a half times to twice as many of the High IQ group in higher socio-economic positions than the moderate IQ group. There would seem to be some perpetuation, at least in expectation, between the three generations in this sample, though doubtless there were individual variations in the pattern across time.

The most conspicuously absent variables were those relating to problem behaviour in the children. High IQ children most certainly did not show problems of sleep, either in disturbance or length of sleep. They were not seen as particularly sensitive or emotional. Above all, they were not seen as 'difficult' children by their parents, who also did not report that these highly intelligent children watched more educational-type television than the more moderately intelligent children. In all, these children seemed to be very well balanced. It was only in their lack of friends that the children's behaviour could be said to be less happy than average, but possibly the children concerned were not perturbed by this situation. Characteristically, the children were doing well at school and the parents were happy about the school.

| The children: understanding | IQ groups | |
|---|---|---|
| | *High* | *Moderate* |
| Can pay attention to more than one thing at once | 43 | 24 |
| The world is sometimes too slow | 30 | 14 |
| Can always understand what other people mean | 24 | 14 |
| | (in percentages of 82 and 128) | |

The High IQ group seemed to have a more flexible and penetrating intellect than the Moderate IQ group. They very often said that they were quite happily able to follow two conversations at once or watch TV and read at the same time. The proportion who said they were able to do this was almost twice that in the Moderate IQ group. Their lively minds caused them some frustration, however, with the normal world - in particular the 'slowness' of other people. From the watcher's point of view, these children may seem to be impatient, but they have often got the point of the argument long before the full explanation has been offered.

To a less significant degree ($p < 0.05$), the High IQ children reported more often than the Moderate IQ children that they could see life through others' eyes, i.e. empathise. This ability to empathise might be considered a personality factor, but it was certainly not pinpointed in the personality tests the children undertook. It was noticeable here, though, in the comparison of intelligence. Also at a less significant level, the High IQ children said they talked a lot, but this idea was not supported by parents or teachers. It was the children's own perception of themselves that they talked more than other children. However, when the children were asked about what people may like or dislike about them, there were no differences between the groups in their replies.

## The children's descriptions of themselves

More significant differences emerged in the comparison between the High and Moderate IQ groups than had been found between the target and control groups. Only those which were significant at the 1% ($p < 0.01$) level are given.

| The children: interests | IQ groups | |
|---|---|---|
| | High | Moderate |
| Many musical interests | 20 | 9 |
| Many cultural or intellectual interests | 35 | 17 |
| Wide variety of interests | 51 | 34 |
| Teacher's personality has no effect on child's learning | 45 | 28 |
| Wide variety of advice for teachers | 39 | 17 |
| High status choice for future occupation | 72 | 59 |
| | (in percentages of 82 and 128) | |

The High IQ children again reflect their parents' leisure patterns. In the first place, they had a considerable interest in musical activities; they were also much more able to play music than the Moderate IQ group and had had more music lessons outside school. But in addition, they showed twice as much interest as the Moderate IQ group in more general intellectual and cultural activities. These activities included dramatic clubs, stamp collecting, 'looking at things', 'making up puzzles', 'making stories from the encyclopaedia' and many more. The High IQ group could be seen to be mentally more active and were curious about most things; they read a lot and made good use of their local library.

Neither group showed more interest in competitive sport than the other. This is in agreement with the parents' descriptions of the High IQ group, i.e. that two-thirds of them were no livelier than other children. There was a somewhat higher proportion of boys in the High IQ group, which could possibly have enhanced their interest in sport, but in fact there was no noticeable difference between the groups in this respect.

As the High IQ group did have many more purposeful activities than the Moderate IQ group, it may be wondered how the latter spent their leisure time. Neither group watched TV more than the other, nor played more sport. Most probably, the Moderate IQ group spent less time on specific activities and more on chatting with friends, reading comics or generally 'hanging around', as children usually do.

The High IQ children were more outspoken about their school lives. They had far more to say about how they should be taught and the kind of teachers they preferred. However, in spite of these stated preferences, they were significantly more independent of the personality of the teacher than the Moderate IQ group, in that almost half of them felt her personality was irrelevant to their learning.

The High IQ children were far more ambitious in their wishes for future occupations than the Moderate IQ group and these could well have been reflected from the societies in which both groups were being brought up. The children's hoped-for occupations were in close correspondence to those of the actual occupations of the fathers of the two groups.

The questionnaire which the children answered was not designed as an 'in-depth' interview, but it did provide some insight into the children's thoughts and feelings.

It looks as though the High IQ children could accept that they were different from other children in terms of their greater amount of talking, but not of any other behaviour. Their thinking was, however, their own business and questions on it could be answered openly. There is undoubtedly a need, felt in the middle years of children, to conform to prevailing behaviour patterns and the High IQ group seemed to adhere to this as closely as their school-mates.

## The teachers

The following is the most dramatic finding of the whole research. On the teachers' reports of the child's behaviour in school, *there was absolutely no difference between the High IQ and Moderate IQ groups*. Close combing of the results of the Bristol Social Adjustment guides did not produce one single behavioural difference, of even low significance, between the High IQ and Moderate IQ groups. There were clearly no differences in the children's observable school behaviour that were due to IQ alone. The behaviour which had distinguished the target children from their controls could not have been due to their IQ difference, but must have been due to some other factors.

It cannot be now said, on the basis of these research findings, that intellectually gifted children are unhappy and show troubled behaviour just because of their gifts. The target children, of undoubtedly high ability, had been compared with controls of similar ability and were seen to behave in a disturbed way. The High IQ group, of even higher ability, when compared to children of moderate ability, were no different in their behaviour.

The target group had formed two-thirds of the High IQ group. It could be expected, therefore, that their disturbing presence would have been effective in the comparisons with the Moderate IQ group, which contained only one-third of their number. There was a possibility that it was the Moderate IQ children in the target group, under pressure from their ambitious parents, who had formed the bulk of the unhappy children.

## Comparison of the High IQ and Moderate IQ children in the original target group

In order to investigate the possibility that the Moderate IQ target children were reacting to pressure from their parents, the target group was divided into High IQ (over 140 IQ) and Moderate IQ (140 and under IQ) groups and compared on all variables. The following variables were all significantly different at 1% ($p < 0.01$).

| *Target group parents* | *Children's IQ scores* | |
|---|---|---|
| | *High* | *Moderate* |
| Mother's high status occupation | 62 | 35 |
| Mothers read a lot | 38 | 22 |
| Mother reads widely | 26 | 17 |
| Child makes excellent school progress | 55 | 17 |
| Child has extraordinary memory | 47 | 26 |
| Child expected to stay in education till 21 years old | 91 | 61 |
| | (in percentages of 47 and 23) | |

The list of variables which distinguished the High IQ and Moderate IQ target children seemed to be a shorter, but typical, selection of those which distinguished between the intelligence groups of the whole population. The children of the target group who had been measured as gifted in IQ emerged from this questionnaire as being in a more favourable educational position than the less able children of the target group. Their mothers enjoyed a higher occupational status and a higher literary level for relaxation. The High IQ children were doing much better at school than the moderately intelligent children and had an exceedingly high level of expected late stay in education. Thus, although the parents of these children of moderate intelligence had all joined the National Association for Gifted Children, the children could be seen to be faring less well than intellectually gifted children in the same association.

At a lower level of significance ($p < 0.05$), the High IQ target children were also found to be heavier at birth, to have read earlier, to have worse handwriting, to have a longer span of concentration and to have received more scholastic help. Their fathers occupied a higher socio-economic occupation than the Moderate IQ group fathers and, like the high IQ mothers, read more.

Most noticeably absent from these comparisons were the parents' descriptions of their children's behaviour problems. There seemed to be no difference in this respect, as far as parents were concerned, whether their children had High or Moderate IQs. The problem behaviour in children appeared to be shared equally across the range of abilities of the target children. There were no differences in the sleep patterns of the High IQ and Moderate IQ target children. As pressure on the children to achieve was similar for both the High IQ and the Moderate IQ target children, the less able children were clearly not reacting to such pressure with behaviour disturbances. The report from the teachers (the BSAG) concurred with this view. There were no differences between the High IQ and Moderate IQ target children with regard to their behaviour in school. The behaviour was spread throughout the group, regardless of their intellectual ability.

When the children's own questionnaire was examined, there proved to be only one very significant difference between the High IQ and Moderate IQ target children. The High IQ children were very much better at paying attention to more than one thing at once. To a lesser degree, the High IQ children read more and found the world too slow for them. There was thus nothing in the children's responses to indicate why some of them showed disturbed behaviour.

## Additional information

Gleaning the responses from parents and teachers had proved to be very informative about the experimental groups. The same procedure was carried out for the IQ groups. The quality of the physical health of the children had been found to be very different between the target and control groups. This was how the adults reported the physical health of the 82 High IQ and 128 Moderate IQ group children, given in percentages of their group numbers.

| Children's physical health | IQ groups | | | |
| --- | --- | --- | --- | --- |
| | High IQ | | Moderate IQ | |
| | Teachers | Parents | Teachers | Parents |
| Stomach complaints | 2 | 2 | 3 | 2 |
| Respiratory/nervous complaints | 12 | 27 | 3 | 18 |
| Speech problems | 12 | 2 | 9 | 2 |
| Poor eyesight | 7 | 0 | 10 | 2 |
| Poor coordination | 6 | 15 | 2 | 2 |
| **Totals** | 39 | 46 | 27 | 26 |
| Average percentages reported | 43 | | 27 | |
| | (in percentages of 82 and 128) | | | |

The differences in the children's physical health, as reported for the High and Moderate IQ groups, was almost identical to that for the target and control groups. The High IQ group had over one and a half times more physical ill-health than the Moderate IQ group. However, these figures cannot be regarded as typical of high IQ children in general; they are specific to this sample. The High IQ group had been composed of well over half of the NAGC children, whose parents had patently sought help for some reason and so were likely to have more than their share of problems.

In order to test this hypothesis – that the target group children had been influential in affecting the comparison of physical health between the High and Moderate IQ groups – they were compared minus the target group children. Thus, children of high and moderate IQ, whose parents had never shown concern about their children's giftedness, were being compared.

| Children's physical health: minus target children | IQ groups | | | |
|---|---|---|---|---|
| | High IQ | | Moderate IQ | |
| | Teachers | Parents | Teachers | Parents |
| Stomach complaints | 2 | 1 | 2 | 1 |
| Respiratory/nervous complaints | 4 | 13 | 2 | 13 |
| Speech problems | 6 | 1 | 7 | 2 |
| Poor eyesight | 2 | 0 | 6 | 2 |
| Poor coordination | 1 | 2 | 1 | 2 |
| **Totals** | 15 | 17 | 18 | 20 |
| Average percentages reported | 16 | | 19 | |

Without the target children, IQ was virtually unrelated to the physical health of the sample. The target children had clearly been responsible for the high figure of physical ill-health among the High IQ group. These aspects of health are usually considered to be indicators of anxiety in children and it may be concluded that the target children did indeed have a higher level of anxiety than either of the control groups. But anxiety was not found to be related to IQ alone.

As there appeared to be a difference in physical attributes between the target and control children, as described by their teachers, this feature was examined for the High and Moderate intelligence groups.

It has often been found in research on gifted children that they are tall for their ages. But it was not found to be so in this study. The reason is probably to do with the social class of the sample population which was, on the whole, very high. Gifted children are often found to be more prevalent among the upper than the lower social levels. By removing this differentiating social factor from the comparison between the measured gifted and the ungifted, IQ on its own was not seen to affect the height of children. But, doubtless, better nourished children are taller and more likely to score well on intelligence tests than smaller, less well nourished children.

| Children's attractiveness | IQ groups | |
|---|---|---|
| | High | Moderate |
| Attractive | 49 | 43 |
| Not so attractive | 11 | 7 |
| | (in percentages of 82 and 128) | |

When the aspect of the children's attractiveness to their teachers had been examined in terms of the experimental groups, there were virtually no differences between them. The comparison of the IQ groups again showed that teachers found children of greater or lesser IQ virtually the same in respect of attractiveness.

| Children's sleep patterns | IQ groups | |
|---|---|---|
| | High | Moderate |
| Disturbed sleep | 24 | 4 |
| Symptoms resulting in disturbed sleep | 12 | 8 |
| | (in percentages of 82 and 128) | |

There had been a highly significant difference between the target and control groups when they had been compared with respect to their sleep patterns, both from the questionnaire material and from parents' remarks – the target children had much poorer quality of sleep. When the IQ groups were compared on the questionnaire material there had been no statistically significant difference between them. The above differences were taken from the additional information given by parents. It seemed that those parents who offered extra information about their children's sleeping habits were those who had something to complain about. It could be expected that when parents were asked if their child had sleep problems and they replied 'no', nothing further was to be said. However, if they answered 'yes' then further explanation seemed to follow which was picked up in this additional perusal of the comments written on the questionnaires.

In order to find out the effect of the target children on the sleep pattern comparisons, the IQ groups were compared minus the target children.

| Children's sleep patterns; minus target children | IQ groups | |
|---|---|---|
| | High | Moderate |
| Disturbed sleep | 4 | 9 |
| Symptoms resulting in disturbed sleep | 2 | 4 |
| | (in percentages of 82 and 128) | |

Without the target children, the High IQ group seemed, if anything, to sleep more soundly than the Moderate IQ group. Again, as with physical health problems, the sleep problems lay clearly with the target group and could not be said to be a function of high IQ alone.

The family backgrounds of the two IQ groups were then examined.

| Unusual home backgrounds | IQ groups | |
|---|---|---|
| | High | Moderate |
| Remarriage | 5 | 5 |
| One-parent family | 5 | 2 |
| Adopted child | 2 | 2 |
| Siblings over eight years older | 2 | 5 |
| | (in percentages of 82 and 128) | |

There was no obvious difference between the family backgrounds of the High and Moderate IQ groups in this direct comparison. But as the original target group had formed two-thirds of the High IQ group and in comparison to its control groups, had shown evidence of unusual family backgrounds, the IQ groups comparison was re-examined minus the target children. The results are given overleaf.

The target families had clearly been affecting the comparisons between the High and Moderate IQ groups in terms of their family composition. Without this original number, the children of the High IQ group were seen to come from more stable backgrounds than those of the Moderate IQ group. The virtual absence of High IQ children with much older siblings was surprising, as it is often thought that children born much later than others in the family are more like first born children and could be expected to have a higher level of intelligence. But it does not appear to be so for this sample at least.

| Unusual home backgrounds: minus the target children | IQ groups | |
|---|---|---|
| | High | Moderate |
| Remarriage | — | 4 |
| One-parent family | — | 1 |
| Adopted child | 1 | 2 |
| Siblings over eight years older | 1 | 5 |
| | (in percentages of 82 and 128) | |

A high proportion of the NAGC parents were teachers. This finding could have been due to a primary concern with educational matters for their children, whether these were gifted or not. Analysis of the number of teachers among parents in terms of the IQ groups gave the following results:

| Parents who are teachers | IQ groups | |
|---|---|---|
| | High | Moderate |
| Only mother teachers | 15 | 12 |
| Only father teachers | 5 | 2 |
| Both parents teach | 12 | 4 |
| Percentage of children with teacher parents | 32 | 18 |
| | (in percentages of 82 and 128) | |

The biggest difference between the IQ groups was where both parents taught. It would be possible to deduce that when both parents are teachers, the child has a higher likelihood of scoring well on an intelligence test. If only one parent teaches, it doesn't seem to make any difference. However, this is only a small sample and a wider study would be needed to validate this particular finding.

## Summary of the IQ groups

The original target sample of children had been chosen essentially on the basis of their parents' belief in their giftedness, the criterion being whether they had joined the National Association for Gifted Children. In order to see whether children and their families were actually different in respect of the children's measured IQ, the target children and their controls were regrouped into High IQ and Moderate IQ categories. High IQ was defined as a score between 141 and 170 IQ, while the moderate category was composed of all the children in the sample with scores below that, which varied between 97 and 140 IQ.

Many significant differences were found in the home backgrounds of the High and Moderate IQ groups. Mothers and fathers of the High IQ group not only had highly intelligent children, but very high status occupations, high levels of education, were avid readers and had a wide variety of interests. They were not dissatisfied with their lively and comfortable lives. These parents were very helpful to their children's scholastic careers in terms of both provision and encouragement. They were also keen on including aesthetics in their children's education and generally expected them to stay in full-time education till after the age of 21.

The High IQ group homes were organized around the hearing and practice of music to a far greater extent than the Moderate IQ homes. Their standard of literature was higher and of a wider variety; they were also situated in better class neighbourhoods. The picture of the high IQ child's home was that of a detached house in a pleasant suburb, the house lined with books and bathed in the sounds of music.

There were only two distinct differences (both verbal) between IQ groups in the children's development, as reported by their parents. The High IQ group children talked and read much earlier than the Moderate IQ group children. But then the test with which their IQs had been measured did have a verbal bias (p. 104). The High IQ group children were not seen by their parents as more alert at birth, nor were there more first born and only children among them than in the Moderate IQ group.

When the parents described their children's behaviour, problems were noticeably absent as features of either group. The High IQ group children were seen as very lively and independent; they possessed extraordinary memories and could concentrate for great lengths of time. They were making excellent progress at school, though their handwriting tended to be poor. The High IQ group children did not

*191*

have many friends and those that they had tended to be older than themselves; their parents described them as 'feeling different'. Like their parents, they were avid readers with a wide variety of interests.

The children described themselves in a similar way to their parents' perception of them. High IQ children were lively with a wide range of interests, but did not see themselves as 'different' from other children. They felt themselves to be relatively independent of the various styles of teaching that they might receive. A high proportion of them wanted a high status occupation. High IQ children were more able to divide their attention and seemed to think far more quickly than other children; they were also able to comprehend meanings more easily.

As far as the class teachers were concerned, there were absolutely no differences in the social classroom behaviour of the High and Moderate IQ groups. Clearly, there were no differences in respect of adjustment in school which were due to IQ alone. It cannot be said that intellectually gifted children are unhappy and show troubled behaviour in a non-specialist school, just because of their intellectual gifts. The teachers did not find the higher IQ children more attractive than the children of moderate IQ.

The High IQ group children were found to be in better physical health and slept more soundly than the Moderate IQ group children. Their family backgrounds were also more stable. More of the High IQ group children had parents who were teachers.

In the comparisons of the experimental groups, parents of the target children described significantly more behaviour problems in their children than had either of the two control groups' parents. To see whether these problems had any relationship to measured IQ within the target group, those 70 children were compared on the basis of their IQ scores. Target children of 141 IQ or more were compared on all the data with target children of 140 IQ or less.

The differences between the high and moderate IQ target children were very similar to those found when the whole sample was compared for IQ. In particular, the high IQ target children had mothers in better social and educational positions. The childen had outstanding memories, were doing well at school and were almost all expected to stay in full-time education till they were 21 years old. Behaviour problems in the target children were to be found across the whole IQ range. Thus, their behaviour problems were not due to the singular effects of IQ, but had other independent or combined origins.

# THE ADJUSTMENT GROUPS

The search was now on for those children whose parents and teachers had described them as showing problem behaviour. They had been seen as forming a large part of the original target group. However, enquiry into the possible effects of ability had demonstrated that this difficult behaviour was independent of measured IQ for this population.

The whole sample was therefore examined with regard to the behaviour of the children in school, the criterion used being each child's score on the Bristol Social Adjustment Guides (BSAG), (Stott, 1976). The class teachers provided the information on these Guides, obtained systematically with regard to all aspects of the child's behaviour in school. As parents and teachers had been in general agreement on which children were troublesome, this teachers' score considered to be representative of parents' opinions.

The range of BSAG scores which were given to this sample provided a basis for redividing the children once again into comparative groups. The scores varied from 0, indicating good adjustment, to 41, which described very poor adjustment, although children who had very high scores were very few in number. The new groupings of children were those of Good, Moderate or Poor adjustment in terms of this sample. The cut-off points which were used to form the adjustment groups were as follows:

| Adjustment group | BSAG scores | Number of children |
|---|---|---|
| Poor | 12 or more | 25 |
| Moderate | 3-11 | 88 |
| Good | 2 or less | 97 |

Each of these groups was compared to the other two on all the data.

As it had been the target children who appeared to be so poorly adjusted in comparison with their controls, the original experimental groups were re-examined in terms of the adjustment groups. The figures given overleaf are the percentages of all the children in the three adjustment groups, rounded off to the nearest whole number.

By far the largest proportion of children (64%) in the composition of the Poor Adjustment group were from the original target group; this is eight times the proportion of children from the control-one group, matched on ability. The Moderate Adjustment group contained about the same proportion of children from each of the three original experimental groups. But there were about half as many target group children as control children in the Good Adjustment group. This was further confirmation of the evidence, described earlier, that target children were less well adjusted than the control children. But a further breakdown of these 25 poorly adjusted children was needed.

| Experimental groups | Adjustment groups | | |
|:---:|:---:|:---:|:---:|
| | Poor | Moderate | Good |
| T | 64 | 38 | 22 |
| $C_1$ | 8 | 33 | 40 |
| $C_2$ | 28 | 30 | 38 |
| | (in percentages of 25, 88 and 97) | | |

## The Poor Adjustment group

The next move was to examine the Poor Adjustment group children in terms of their measured IQ, lest there be any possibility of a connection between IQ and behaviour disturbance. They were also re-examined in terms of the original experimental groups. This produced a clear picture, given below in percentages of the 25 children:

| Poor adjustment group | T | $C_1$ | $C_2$ | Totals |
|:---|:---:|:---:|:---:|:---:|
| High IQ | 40 | 0 | 0 | 40 |
| Moderate IQ | 24 | 8 | 28 | 60 |
| Totals | 64 | 8 | 28 | 100 |
| | | (in percentages of 25) | | |

It was only in the target group that High IQ seemed to be in any way related to poor adjustment. There were twice as many High IQ target children as Moderate IQ target children in the Poor Adjustment category. The absence of poorly adjusted High IQ children in both control groups, however, strengthened the idea that IQ was not in itself a prerequisite for difficult behaviour. Of all the children in the Poor Adjustment group, 60% were of moderate ability. The Average IQ levels for the three groups were:

| Poor Adjustment | 148.8 |
|---|---|
| Moderate Adjustment | 141.5 |
| Good Adjustment | 151.6 |

These figures are not significantly different and, by their very similarity, demonstrate again that High IQ and societal maladjustment are not related.

## Home background

There is a contemporary tendency to place the blame (rarely the praise) for children's behaviour squarely on the parents, viz. 'There are no difficult children; only difficult parents'. It was possible that the poorly adjusted group would be found to have had different parenting from that of the other two adjustment groups.

In fact, there were remarkably few differences in the home backgrounds of the three adjustment groups and those that did emerge were not statistically significant ($p < 0.05$). The mothers of the Good Adjustment group read more than the other mothers and the parents of this group gave their children more scholastic attention than those of the other groups. However, fathers of the Poor Adjustment group were somewhat less satisfied with their educations than those of the other adjustment groups. Parents were also more likely to give the Poor Adjustment group children presents, rather than praise, as a reward.

The big differences between the groups were in the parents' descriptions of their children. They are given below in percentages of the adjustment groups. Only those variables which showed significant differences between the groups at the 1% level ($p < 0.01$) are presented.

| Children's behaviour: parents' description | Adjustment groups | | |
|---|---|---|---|
| | Poor | Moderate | Good |
| Very 'difficult' | 28 | 10 | 6 |
| Feels 'different' | 52 | 23 | 7 |
| Poor work in school | 48 | 25 | 14 |
| School progress poor | 16 | 6 | 4 |
| Handwriting poor | 40 | 30 | 18 |
| | (in percentages of 25, 88 and 97) | | |

The most striking aspect of this list of variables, which distinguished between the adjustment groups at home, was the absence of those behaviour problems that the target parents had spoken about. The Poor Adjustment group were not described by their parents as particularly sensitive, very emotional, independent of mind or having problems with sleep more frequently than the better adjusted groups. The teachers had described these children as being very difficult in the classroom and the parents seemed to have 'underlined' that statement. They were in entire agreement with the teachers that the children's work in school was poor and that the children had problems in coping with life.

The statement on which parents and teachers were in undoubted agreement was that the child was 'difficult', but there may have been some difference of opinion as to what defined a child as difficult. The parents' concerns were with problematical behaviour of everyday life, while the children who were selected by teachers as being difficult showed problematical behaviour in school. Unfortunately, the questions asked of both sets of adults could not be the same; for example, the teachers would find it difficult to describe the sleeping habits of their pupils. However, there was clear agreement between parents and teachers about the children who were not doing well at school. Of the poorly adjusted children, 40% were of High IQ and their apparently distressed parents had all joined the association for gifted children. It was not surprising that parents described their children as feeling 'different' since they *were* actually different from their schoolmates. Many of them had the treble distinction of being intellectually gifted and out of sympathy with both school and parents.

There were other aspects of the children's behaviour which were less significant ($p < 0.05$) but which added to the same picture. The Poor Adjustment group were the least selective in the type of television they watched while the Good Adjustment group were more likely to know which programmes they wanted and when they were being shown. The Poor Adjustment group were less persevering than the better adjusted children; they seemed to be less able to grasp a problem and wrestle with it.

The Poor Adjustment group were more likely to have attended nursery school, but the reasons for this must remain speculative. As they had been described as difficult, this could have been a move by the parents towards tranquillity in the home. Perhaps it was hoped that their time spent in the organized life of a nursery would ease the transition to school. But any form of early socialization process with these children was clearly less than successful. Their behaviour in the classroom was not acceptable to their teachers and they were not very popular with their schoolmates, as they were unlikely to have many friends. The friends which they did have were neither older nor younger, merely scarce. Their original position in the family seemed to have some relevance to their unhappiness, as the Poor Adjustment group were more likely to be first born or only children than those in the other groups.

## The children

There were no significant differences between the children of the various adjustment groups when they were compared on their self-descriptions. Whatever strong words the adults who look after them may find to use about them, it is probable that the children do not wish to distinguish themselves from other children in terms of unacceptable (to adults) behaviour.

The personality questionnaires (see p. 137) which had been given to the whole sample had failed to throw light on any personality differences between the various groups under comparison. However, there was one highly significant personality difference between the Poor and Good Adjustment group. The less well adjusted children appeared as being considerably more 'warmhearted' – more out-going and participating – whereas the better adjusted children were decidedly more 'reserved', i.e. more detached and aloof. It may be that there is a price to be paid for teacher approval, which is something like a dampening of the spirit.

## The teachers

The important differences between the three adjustment groups, as reported by the teachers, are all concerned with aspects of the children's over-reaction. The variables presented below are all significantly different ($p < 0.01$) between the Poor and Good Adjustment groups. They are the percentages of children in each adjustment group who were scored at all for each category. This information is more precise than the description of poor general adjustment; it shows just what the teachers were complaining about. In the Poor Adjustment group, their greatest problem was their tendency to show-off, closely followed by their inability to keep still. They were easily distracted, moody or sullen and attention-seeking. The Good Adjustment group showed only a tiny percentage of these problem behaviours.

| Details of over-reaction | Adjustment groups | | |
|---|---|---|---|
| | Poor | Moderate | Good |
| Inconsequence | | | |
| Distractable | 56 | 10 | — |
| Hyperactive | 68 | 26 | 4 |
| Showing off | 72 | 23 | 3 |
| Attention-seeking | 44 | 22 | 9 |
| Hostility | | | |
| Moody/sullen | 56 | 23 | 3 |
| | | (in percentages of 25, 88 and 97) | |

## Additional information

The same gleaning of parents' and teachers' responses was carried out for the adjustment groups as had been done for the experimental and IQ groups. This was of material from the questionnaires which had not been pre-rated.

The children's physical health could have been of considerable importance in their adjustment. Stott (1976) has said that unhealthy children showed up as less well adjusted than healthy children on his guides.

| Children's physical health | Adjustment groups | | | | | |
|---|---|---|---|---|---|---|
| | Poor | | Moderate | | Good | |
| | Teachers | Parents | Teachers | Parents | Teachers | Parents |
| Stomach complaints | 0 | 4 | 6 | 2 | 3 | 1 |
| Respiratory complaints | 20 | 24 | 6 | 22 | 4 | 21 |
| Speech problems | 24 | 0 | 11 | 2 | 6 | 2 |
| Poor eyesight | 0 | 0 | 11 | 0 | 9 | 2 |
| Poor co-ordination | 12 | 8 | 6 | 11 | 1 | 3 |
| **Totals** | 56 | 36 | 40 | 37 | 23 | 29 |
| Average percentage reported | 46 | | 39 | | 26 | |
| | | | | (in percentages of 25, 88 and 97) | | |

As children were measured in terms of their diminishing adjustment, so they appeared to be less physically fit. The biggest difference in health was between children who had been scored as poorly adjusted and those scored as well adjusted. The Poor Adjustment group had nearly twice as many afflictions as the Good Adjustment group. They seemed to be particularly prone to respiratory complaints and had a high proportion of speech problems.

The data were examined to determine how the children, who had been scored by their teachers for behaviour in class, were seen by them in terms of attractiveness.

| Children's attractiveness | Adjustment groups | | |
|---|---|---|---|
| | Poor | Moderate | Good |
| Attractive | 28 | 35 | 59 |
| Not so attractive | 12 | 14 | 3 |
| | (in percentages of 25, 88 and 97) | | |

There appeared to be a fairly direct relationship between adjustment score and the attractiveness of the child; the better adjusted the child, the more attractive he appeared. This is not entirely surprising as a maladjusted child could not be expected to be as attractive to a teacher as a well adjusted child. But in spite of this, nearly a third of the poor adjustment group *were* described as attractive.

It would be expected that children with behaviour problems would have accompanying sleep problems. This was the picture for sleep in relation to the adjustment groups:

| Children's sleep patterns | Adjustment groups | | |
|---|---|---|---|
| | Poor | Moderate | Good |
| Disturbed sleep | 40 | 16 | 11 |
| Symptoms resulting in disturbed sleep | 24 | 10 | 6 |
| | (in percentages of 25, 88 and 97) | | |

A similar relationship was found to that between the attractiveness of the children and their social adjustment scores. The more maladjusted the child, the worse his sleep pattern. Of the 39 parents who said their children had disturbed sleep, 24 were target parents.

The home circumstances of the children could reasonably be expected to affect their adjustment in school. The relationship of unusual home background to the adjustment group was as follows:

| Unusual home background | Adjustment groups | | |
|---|---|---|---|
| | Poor | Moderate | Good |
| Remarriage | 0 | 9 | 3 |
| One-parent family | 12 | 2 | 1 |
| Adopted child | 8 | 3 | 0 |
| Siblings over 8 years old | 0 | 9 | 2 |
| | (in percentages of 25, 88 and 97) | | |

The unusualness of the home background appeared to be influential in the children's behaviour in a two-way split. Relatively few of the children of the Good Adjustment group had unusual home backgrounds, but those of either the Moderate or Poor Adjustment groups did. The poorest adjustment was found in the children of one-parent families and those lone parents were also the ones who had most frequently sought help from the NAGC.

It was interesting to see whether there was any relationship between the children's adjustment scores in school and their parents being teachers:

| Parents who are teachers | Adjustment groups | | |
|---|---|---|---|
| | Poor | Moderate | Good |
| Only mother teaches | 12 | 15 | 6 |
| Only father teaches | 4 | 3 | 3 |
| Both parents teach | 4 | 7 | 8 |
| | (in percentages of 25, 88 and 97) | | |

Having teachers as parents does not, on the whole, seem to be detrimental to the child's adjustment. However, there was a higher percentage of poorly adjusted children when only the mother taught, compared to when only the father or both parents taught. I can offer no reasonable explanation for such a revelation.

## Boys and girls

Of the 25 children in the poorly adjusted group, 19 (76%) were boys and six (24%) were girls. As this represented a much higher proportion of boys to girls than in the total sample, there was the possibility that boys were being regarded as difficult more often than girls. In fact, boys are often seen by teachers as being less conforming than girls, particularly at primary school. Perhaps they are being unfairly picked on; much American educational literature has described how boys suffer from an overwhelmingly female teaching force in the primary school. These schoolmarms are said to dampen the boy's spirit of adventure, to narrow his thinking and to offer no change from Mom. As girls theoretically have no problems of identification, being of the same sex as their mothers and teachers, they do not appear to suffer from these restrictions. The boys might have been rebelling against continued female authority and were being regarded unfavourably by their mentors as a result.

The children of the Poor Adjustment group were considered in terms of their sex and IQ.

| Poor adjustment | Boys | Girls |
|---|---|---|
| High IQ | 32 | 8 |
| Moderate IQ | 44 | 16 |
| | (in percentages of 25) | |

Again there was no evidence that high IQ promoted poor adjustment; in fact the opposite conclusion could be drawn, i.e. that a higher IQ brought about better adjustment than a lesser IQ. However, there was a higher proportion of boys to girls for both of the IQ ranges in the Poor Adjustment group.

An investigation was also made into whether the children were taught by members of their own sex or not and no significant difference was found in the sex of the teacher for boys or girls. There were probably two reasons for this. Firstly, that many more men now teach in English primary schools than even a few years ago; one or two men teachers are usually to be found in any primary school. Secondly, there was a high proportion (43%) of private schools in this sample. Such schools in

England are most often single-sex schools, even at primary level. Statistically each child was very likely to be taught by a teacher of the same sex and therefore the boys' scores on the BSAG were unlikely to be affected overall by a preponderance of female teachers. Stott (1976) estimated that between 11–15% of boys and 8% of girls are maladjusted in Britain. The proportions of the two sexes showing maladjustment in this sample were similar.

The problem behaviour which the boys showed more than the girls was all in the category of 'over-reactive'. These boys were more attention-seeking and less able to make friends, but, above all, were generally less self-controlled than the girls.

## Summary of the adjustment groups

These new regroupings were made on the basis of the child's total score on the Bristol Social Adjustment Guide. This was a report by the teachers of the child's behaviour in class, and was in agreement with the parents' report from home. Comparisons were made between the Poor, Moderate and Good Adjustment groups on all the data to seek possible causes for their patterns of behaviour.

The largest proportion (64%) of children in the Poor Adjustment group were from the original target group. An investigation of the children's IQs in this Poor Adjustment group showed that the target children also provided all the high IQ children (40%) in it. The other 60% of children in the Poor Adjustment group were of moderate IQ. In fact there was no significant difference in IQ across the three adjustment groups. Yet again, IQ was seen to be ineffective as a source of potential maladjustment.

There were few differences in the home backgrounds of children in the three adjustment groups. To a moderate extent, the parents of the Good Adjustment group gave their children more scholastic encouragement and read more themselves. Parents of the Poor Adjustment group were more inclined to give their children presents rather than praise for rewards and fathers were less satisfied with their educations.

The Poor Adjustment group parents described their children as significantly more difficult to bring up and as feeling 'different' much more often. Not surprisingly perhaps, the Poor Adjustment group were not doing well at school and also had poor handwriting. There were only ten children (12.2% of the High IQ group) who were not doing well scholastically and who were ill-adjusted. All their parents had joined the National Association for Gifted Children.

Other less significant features of the Poor Adjustment children were that they seemed less able to organize themselves. They tended to watch television indiscriminately and to give up a problem more easily. Their friends were few in number and they were more likely to be first-born or only children. More of them had been to nursery school than children in the better adjusted groups.

When asked about themselves, the children did not perceive themselves as different. The personality tests showed them to be more outgoing and participating than the other groups. Their teachers, however, found them to be particularly over-reactive. They tended to draw attention to themselves, particularly by running around the classroom. They were easily distracted in lessons and were of a moody or sullen disposition.

The physical health of the Poor Adjustment group was worse than that of the better adjusted groups having nearly twice as many afflictions, particularly respiratory complaints and speech problems.

Teachers described the children as more attractive the better adjusted they were. The same relationship was found between adjustment and sleep patterns – the worse the adjustment, the more likely the children were to have sleep disturbances.

Where home circumstances were unusual, they did appear to affect the children. Those of the Moderate and Poor adjustment groups came from less stable homes than the children of the Good Adjustment group. The least well adjusted children were found in one-parent families.

A further investigation into whether the sex of the children was likely to affect their adjustment score on these guides was negative. Boys were not seen as more deviant than girls by their teachers. In this sample, children of either sex were most likely to be taught by a teacher of their own sex.

## THE SCHOOLS

The first selection of children in this research had been from the records of the National Association for Gifted Children. Each of these target children was allotted two control children from the same school class. Accordingly, the schools which each triad attended formed the sample of schools; these numbered 61 and were of many kinds, spread over the North West of England.

By selecting the control children from the same school class, the three experimental groups were as well matched for educational experience as is possible between human subjects. In addition, as there were no boarding schools involved in the research, the children would normally be drawn from the same school catchment area. The socio-economic environments of each triad would then be similar and differences which arose between each of the three experimental groups of children and families would stand out more clearly from the societal background. This benefit could be seen, for example, when the target group children were compared to the control children and found to be more unhappy. As each of the triads of children were in the same class, in 61 schools, it could not be said that individual schools were in any way responsible for the target group's behaviour in this respect. The causes had to be found elsewhere.

It has often been said by educationalists that gifted children are likely to suffer in the normal classroom. The fear is expressed that, should they be frustrated and 'unstretched', they will make mischief and may turn to crime, as though gifted children were morally more delicate than ordinary children. However, this fear is quite unfounded on any evidence.

In this research, many gifted children were seen, in a wide variety of schools, none of which used specially designed materials or teaching programmes for gifted pupils. The project was designed to look at these children in their social and psychological settings, rather than to examine their educational progress. Consequently, the children were not tested for their level of achievement in any particular subjects. Such a measurement, across this great variety of schools and ages, would have been of doubtful validity in any case.

The variation of schools in England is considerable. Those in this sample ranged from a tiny convent school with 20 pupils to the highly selective Manchester Grammar School with 1500 pupils. Some schools were strongly religious, some were devoted to preparing young boys for expensive private schools and one was for musically gifted children. There were some which accepted children for the whole span of their time in school, while others only took pupils for two or more years. Added to this, there were different age divisions between schools in different local education authorities. Though the ages of the children in the schools listed below overlap to some extent, this simplified presentation does give an idea of the types of schools involved.

Because of the way in which this sample was collected, it did not form a typical group of English schools. The headteachers of each school had been asked to say from which social class the school drew its pupils and, on their estimation, 18% of the schools were upper or middle class, 73% were mixed and only 10% were working-class.

| School | Age range (years) | Numbers of triads |
|---|---|---|
| Infant | 5.00 – 7.11 | 20 |
| Junior | 8.0 – 10.11 | 32 |
| Middle/Secondary | 11.0 – 13.11 | 18 |

As described earlier, the parents of the sample children were of a preponderantly high socio-economic level. They could choose to live in the more attractive districts of their locality or close to the school of their choice, or to pay for a private school. In fact, 43% of these schools were private which is very high in comparison with the national average of 6% private schools.

There was the possibility at the outset of the research that when the target children were found to be gifted, it would have been impossible to match them for ability within their own school class since gifted children are statistically very rare in any country. A fall-back system of cross-school matching was therefore devised. Fortunately, however, it proved to be quite unnecessary and the children were able to be matched with considerable accuracy in their own school class on the Raven's Matrices raw scores.

Part of the reason for this was that the target children were not all gifted. But more importantly, it is a feature of human life that people of a like kind tend to come together and the school catchment area obviously affects the type of children going to that school. In this sample, analysis in terms of social class and IQ resulted in the following pattern. The percentage figures are in terms of the IQ group of the children:

| School area | High IQ children | Moderate IQ children |
|---|---|---|
| Middle class | 32 | 15 |
| Mixed class | 67 | 72 |
| Working class | 5 | 11 |
| | (in percentages 82 and 128) | |

There was a considerable difference in the proportion of High IQ children between middle class and working class schools. Nearly a third

205

of all the High IQ group were in middle class schools and only a twentieth were in working class ones. But there was very little difference between the middle and working class schools in their enrolment of the Moderate IQ children. Children of High IQ did appear to cluster in schools which drew on predominantly middle-class backgrounds. However, there were two gifted children in a school which drew (in the headteacher's words) 'entirely from two municipal housing estates – first or second generation from slum clearance areas'. A target mother described her son's school as 'run down and in a poor area'; she added that the researcher 'would be hard put to find a child as clever as hers in the same class'. She was wrong, however.

## The headteachers

The research did not try to investigate details of the headteachers' private lives, but they were kind enough to provide us with their names and a description of how they set about running their schools. It was not difficult, though, to decide whether they were male or female, which provided some informative comparisons.

Of the 61 headteachers involved in the project, 74% were men and 26% were women; a ratio of 3:1. Even in the infant schools, there were nearly twice as many male headteachers as women. But of the class teachers of the sample children, 26% were men and 74% were women; a ratio of 1:3. This was an extraordinarily exact reversal of proportions; the sex of the rank and file teachers in this sample was thus in directly inverse proportion to the sex of the headteachers. The effect of such a reversal can only be a matter of supposition though.

## The headteacher's concerns

All the headteachers were asked in a questionnaire to describe their school as well as their ideas on education in general and on gifted children in particular. As might have been expected with such a varied group of schools, the headteachers' opinions were also very varied. But, at all times, the headteachers were very sympathetic to the developmental needs of children and were not at all concerned about their social class. Headteachers were particularly concerned about the child's own attitude to education – not that of the parents. They felt that a positive approach was essential to an experience of lifelong significance such as education and tried to promote this in school. Where the headteachers did have clear objectives in education, they seemed to be determined to see them through.

Gifted children were not always seen as a problem by the headteachers. As one said, 'They are as problematic as any other child'. The heads' responses to two specific statements on this subject were as follows (in percentages of all the headteachers):

|                                | *Yes* | *Unsure* | *No* |
|--------------------------------|-------|----------|------|
| Gifted children –              |       |          |      |
| are a problem                  | 44    | 0        | 56   |
| need special education         | 59    | 7        | 34   |
|                                |       |          | (in percentages of 61) |

This sample of headteachers was most certainly biased towards the problems, or the supposed problems, of gifted children. After all, they had been largely selected by parents who believed their children to be gifted. But an average selection of schools from the same area could not be expected to answer even as affirmatively as this one that gifted children posed problems. When asked about how they coped with gifted children, nearly all the headteachers said that they fitted them in with the class teaching, which was geared to the individual children's abilities. One headmaster said, 'Clever children are moved about their age-group'. Another said 'Happiness is the natural corollary to success' and worked on that.

Although most of the headteachers were concerned about children's developmental problems, they were not always very keen to have regular contact with parents. This can be seen primarily in the formal relationships between home and school, as follows (in percentages of the 61 schools):

| A parent–teacher association | 55% |
|------------------------------|-----|
| A parents' association       | 12% |
| No formal relationships      | 33% |

A parent–teacher association raises funds for the school and provides a basis of regular meetings between teachers and those parents who want to come. A parent's association, on the other hand, only raises funds for the school. It is not normal in England for parents to be actively involved in the practice of education in schools. Mothers may sometimes help in infant schools or a parent may come in occasionally to give a talk or demonstration, but participation in curriculum planning is extremely rare. In this sample, only one headteacher of a primary school stated that parents participated in teaching.

Sometimes the headteacher explained that an association was not needed because the school was open to parents and the teachers were always available. Occasionally, this was so: parents wandered in at will and school was like home; but in some schools, it did not seem to be true. For example, mothers would wait for their children very obviously outside the school gates; even when it was pouring with rain, they stood outside and were not invited into the shelter of the school. One headmaster of a private junior school put it very succinctly in heavy capital letters at the end of this questionnaire: 'I would no more dream of allowing a parent to help run my school than I would dream of offering advice to my doctor, solicitor, accountant or any man possessing a profession which I do not have'. He provided boy/father camps, while mothers were not referred to; the school doors were kept locked, but someone would answer the bell. This was presumably the attitude which the parents preferred and were prepared to pay for.

Several headteachers of schools without a formal association explained that teachers were available, but by appointment only. One headmaster went on to say that 'Parent representation on the Governing Body should be sufficient. Parents have access to the head and staff at all times' – but always by appointment. A headmistress claimed that 'her' parents were 'too busy (or contented) to respond' to her suggestion of a parents' association.

The headteachers were asked what they thought about psychological counselling help, which is not normally available in English schools and certainly not in junior schools. They were split in their opinions about this; 51% thought they could use it, 41% were against the idea and 10% didn't know. This was a difference in attitude towards counselling from that found by myself in previous research (Freeman, 1973); then, the great majority of secondary school teachers in the same area, when asked about their feelings towards prospective school counsellors, were dead against the idea.

A school psychological service is available to teachers for those pupils who need it, but the educational psychologists have a very heavy work load and there are often waiting lists. One headmaster was very clear in his feelings about psychological intervention. 'If psychological help means psychologically trained – then no. If it means a friendly and trusted psychiatrist – then yes'. Generally, headteachers seemed to feel that they could handle the problems of gifted or other children by themselves. When the headteachers were asked directly whether teachers could cope with psychological problems, 69% said they could, 3% didn't know and only 28% said that some professional help would be valuable.

An example of current practice in the psychological field was the response to the question of what the head would do if a child was unhappy with his class teacher; 41% said they would transfer the child to another teacher, 3% didn't know, but 56% said that the child would have to stay in that situation. One headmaster of a junior school of 580 pupils said, 'If one child is transferred, others would have be be given the same opportunity and this would make an impossible situation in a school such as this'. Apart from its larger size, it was not apparent how this school was fundamentally different from other junior schools.

Of the 61 schools, only eight were selective; one selected on musical ability and seven on academic ability by means of examinations taken at eleven years old. The seven schools were all ex-Direct Grant schools, i.e. those schools which used to have most of their funds provided directly by the central government, but which were otherwise independent. During the course of this research, their grants were stopped and they became privately funded; this change swelled the number of 'private' schools in the sample. In a sense, gifted children are specially catered for in selective schools; these are not specifically described as being for the gifted but their intake of pupils is of very highly able children, many of whom are gifted. The teaching procedures are not normally different from those in other secondary schools, except of course in the case of the music school. However, the level at which the teachers in these schools can direct their lessons is higher. Even though their children attended such schools, parents who joined the National Association for Gifted Children, by this action alone, expressed a need for some other facilities for their children. In one of these selective schools the pupils had an average IQ of 144, in another the school was devoted to gifted musicians.

Although 87% of the schools were non-selective in intake, 72% of schools divided the children by ability for teaching; 34% did it only for certain subjects, but 56% kept the children in ability classes for all subjects. Nearly all the secondary schools were streamed for ability, as were a few of the junior schools. The amount of ability streaming in a school was related to the size of the school ($r = 0.501$).

Only 20% of the schools were designated as being of a specific religion, but many of the other headteachers were very concerned about their pupils' understanding of religious knowledge; 77% of all headteachers said it was important. Every one of the teachers believed that the teaching of moral values was important.

The headteachers who were concerned for the children to move towards autonomy in their school years cared most about the children's happiness, self-expression, social adjustment and leisure activities. When the school was devoted to improving academic achievement, and this included all the selective schools, the headteachers put considerable effort into providing skills for information seeking and were more certain of the authority of the schools.

## State and private schools

The parents in this sample were able to exercise a considerable choice of school. Because of their own high ability, education and expertise they were often able to move into the area where there was a school they liked or else live in an area where there was a preponderance of people like themselves, whose children would be likely to attend the same school. Additionally, many of the parents could afford to opt out of the state system and chose instead to buy their children a private education.

Reasons for choosing a private or state school are both educational and social; the education may be 'better' and the pupils might also meet 'nicer' children. As there were so many private schools in this sample, all the data was examined with regard to this criterion. An investigation was made into the reasons why such a high proportion of parents in this sample chose private schools. There were 26 private schools (42.62%), attended by 78 children (37.14%). The disproportion in percentages is caused by the presence of more than one triad in some schools. There were, in fact, 70 triads of children in 61 schools.

Re-examination of the data on the basis of state and private schools showed that the greatest influence on a child's attendance at a school was his family – essentially his mother. The occupations and educations of the mothers of private school children were significantly higher ($p < 0.01$) than those of the state school children's mothers. There was relatively little difference between the fathers in status and education. One of the most striking aspects of this study is the extent to which mothers have been found to be influential in their children's development, education and expectations.

# Children's social adjustment in school

There was a possibility, when considering reasons why children should go to private schools, that it was the more 'difficult' children who would attend them. When the scores of the Bristol Social Adjustment Guides were examined in this context, very few differences were found, however, and none were significant at $p < 0.01$.

The children in the private schools were seen by their teachers as somewhat more over-reactive than those in the state schools. They tended to show off more and were more attention-seeking. Although they made friends as easily as the children in the state schools, they were less conforming to their peers.

However, when the group of the poorly adjusted children were looked at in terms of their schools, the picture was clearer. Of the 25 children in the 'poor' group, 72% went to state schools and 28% to private schools. Of the whole sample, 37% of children attended private schools so that it looked as though the state schools were getting more than their fair share of poorly adjusted children. Either the private schools were coping better with potentially maladjusted pupils, or their teachers were looking on them with a more kindly eye when filling in the questionnaires.

The poor adjustment group were examined with regard to their IQs and to the type of school the children were in. There was always the possibility that intellectually gifted children in normal state schools were suffering from frustration or isolation. Of the 18 poorly adjusted children in the state schools, nine were of a high IQ and nine were of a moderate IQ. Thus, high IQ of itself could not be said to have affected the behaviour of these children in the state schools. Of the seven poorly adjusted children in the private schools, two were of a High IQ and five of a Moderate IQ. The figures were, by this stage, too small to merit further deciphering.

## The schools

The biggest difference between the outlooks and practices of private and state schools respectively, in this sample, was in the size of their classes.

The average size of class in the private schools was found to be about five children less than in the state schools. But the variation in size in the private schools was greater; although private schools have a reputation for smaller class size than state schools, parents do not always seem to get what they pay for. The only other notably significant difference between the private and state schools was in the numbers of denominational schools. Most of the 12 denominational schools were private, which accounted for this difference.

| Size of class | Private | State |
|---|---|---|
| Mean | 26.20 | 31.26 |
| Standard deviation | 7.20 | 3.120 |

(Significant at $p < 0.01$)

There were four other, less significant differences between the schools. As might be expected, the private school headteachers were more keen for their pupils to have an understanding of religious knowledge. They were also more concerned for pupils to set their own educational goals. The private schools had better relationships between the headteacher and the staff and they were somewhat more likely to be selective. This last was undoubtedly due to the change of status of the Direct Grant schools from state supported to private during the course of the research. There were five ex-Direct Grant schools in the sample.

There were no social class differences in the school populations, as reported by the headteachers. It had been expected that a comparison of state and private education would have shown up social class differences. In this sample, however, the parental population was of such an overall high social level that only six of the 61 schools were described by their headteachers as having generally working class populations.

The supposition that better-off parents are able to exercise more choice of school is borne out by this research. It looked as though these particular parents had decided on schools with similar outlooks, whether they were private or state. Presumably, if parents could find a state school which offered them what they wanted, they were free to accept it and often did so. If not, they were able to find a private school to suit their needs.

Certainly, as far as this sample was concerned, there were no differences in teaching aims or methods between the private and state schools. Judging by the headteachers' responses to the questionnaire, it looked as though they were not prepared to compromise on their teaching beliefs, whichever type of school they were in. When asked to state the particular characteristics of his school, one headmaster wrote 'Very Expensive'. It was impossible to determine, though, whether parents were generally obtaining a 'nicer' type of companion for their child by buying a private education.

## Summary of the schools

There were several main points of view which divided headteachers in respect of the running of their schools. The most frequently held views, particularly amongst the heads of primary schools, seemed to be considerably influenced by educational psychology. This could have been due to the effects of recent teacher training. Teachers' ages were unfortunately not known, but the ones holding these views were certainly teachers of younger children.

All schools offer education, but some headteachers saw it primarily as a means to autonomy for the child, others as a working partnership with the home and others as a stimulant or means to achievement. They were all concerned, however, with what school should mean to pupils.

Headteachers were not noticeably concerned with children's social class and were not unduly worried by their native abilities. Where gifted children were seen as a problem, heads felt they would be better off with some form of special education. But even in this sample of headteachers, which must have been biased towards considering gifted children as problems, less than half of them subscribed to the idea of giftedness as a problem *per se*. Generally, they felt they could cope with the psychological problems arising from this, or any other condition, by themselves and professional psychological help was not always welcome. For 34% of headteachers, even extra educational help for gifted children would also be unwelcome.

Head-parent relationships were not often close and there seemed to be some room for improvement in this respect. Nearly a third of the schools could only be contacted through appointments, made with the school secretary by the parents. This was nearly always with the implicit understanding that the headteacher's permission was sought before contacting the class teacher. This system would restrict the parents to seeking individual help for specific problems and inhibit involvement with the school as a whole. Only 52% of headteachers approved of parents having any say in the running of the school, but 67% of schools had a formal parent-school association. It can be assumed that the 15% of such associations which functioned without the approval of the headteacher were not very effective in influencing school policy. There had been five headteachers who had refused access to the research, all of them in an entirely autocratic manner. The absence of these headteachers from this sample of schools can only have detracted from the picture of authoritarianism which the remaining heads presented.

When parents felt very strongly about the matter of giftedness, in particular that of their own child, they were faced with considerable problems. Most schools were not geared to the concept of giftedness and those that recognized it as a problem, which they would like to do something about, did not have the means to do so. Almost half the headteachers did not approve of parents having any say in the running of the school and the authority of the headteacher in England virtually assumes that he has his own way. Therefore, in order to be effective for any special interest, parents must act outside the educational establishment and are obliged to join together to promote it. As far as this sample was concerned, the National Association for Gifted Children had been formed to cater for the children of parents who believe them to be gifted and in need of something their schools did not appear to offer. Relatively few people who did not have gifted children themselves joined the association for the benefit of gifted children in general.

The parents in this sample had clearly exercised their ability to choose their child's school. 42.62% of the schools in this sample were private. The greatest influence on this choice was found to come from the mother and was primarily associated with her occupational status and education.

The behaviour of the children in the private and state schools was found to be little different. Those in private schools were marginally more attention-seeking. Relatively more of the less well adjusted children went to state schools, but there was no relationship found between their abilities, supposed frustration and consequent misbehaviour.

Private schools were found to have more variation in class size, and more denominational schools. They seemed to have better relationships within the staff than state schools, but not better parent–teacher relationships. However there were no differences in teaching aims or methods to be found between the differently financed schools. Teachers seemed to teach in the manner which they believed to be right, whatever the characteristics of the school.

# CHAPTER 5

# Gifted Children in Perspective

In seeking a cause for personal troubles in terms of social structures, a complex series of links are found between economic, cultural and political organizations, binding the lives of particular individuals with these wider systems. By demonstrating connections between the stereotype of the 'gifted child' and his social context, we are in a stronger and more informed position from which to take any necessary action. In order to find out whether life events are of causal importance in the physical and mental behaviour of gifted children, it is necessary to show that such behaviour is more frequently found in gifted children of certain environments than others. Comparison groups from the same school population but different home environments provided a basis for the design of my research.

The purpose of the study, described in the previous chapter, was to look at children who were believed by their parents to be gifted. Since its approach was that of social psychology, the design necessarily had to take a double standpoint. The first was inwards from the societal context to see how that affects members of a particular society; the second was outwards from the individuals, to see how they react to the society they live in. Thus, the social milieu of the parents would affect the way they thought about their children and what they valued in them. But at the same time, individual reactions within society would also influence their hopes and expectations for the children.

It was a matter of concern in this study to make findings generally applicable, at least to England. Pilot comparison had shown that there were no statistically significant differences between two quarters of the country – the South-East and the North-West. Since the latter was more convenient, it was chosen as the survey area and the results from it were considered valid for both. As the remaining half of the country would be unlikely to be quite different in these respects, it too would be expected to show the same general picture in an investigation of this kind. Thus the findings of this project are considered to be generally valid throughout England.

## REVIEW OF THE RESEARCH

The variety of ability among gifted children is immense. This research has been restricted largely to gifted children of high IQ because that was how the parents of the target children perceived them. This definition of giftedness is often used for practical purposes, not only in schools but also by psychologists in child guidance clinics. Naturally, there is an intimate connection between the description of giftedness as used in any piece of research and the characteristics of the gifted children under that investigation. It is recognized that if, for instance, gifted artists had been investigated in this research, their characteristics and those of their homes would probably have differed from the ones shown by the high IQ gifted children. The selection of children believed by their parents to be gifted was made on the criterion of parents' recent membership of The National Association for Gifted Children. This was straightforward, as there cannot be borderline cases of membership. Virtually all the parents had joined because of their children's supposed intellectual giftedness. Each of these target children was matched with two control children, the first being of the same intellectual ability, but the second chosen at random from the same school class.

In asking people about the way they live, the questioner is always receiving a personal perspective. The meanings which a father imputes to his child's behaviour or to events in the family are a part of his whole perception of life. But by recording what people actually said, as well as their contexts, the research had a structure in which personal feelings could be placed. For example, a mother may have said that she felt bitter about her past education and yet be a graduate, while another mother who felt satisfied about her education may have left school at the age of 15. The mother's feelings must be seen in the context of her life events. Her subjective experience of education is an influence in her attitudes to it equally important to the number of years she spent in educational establishments. The questionnaires for the parents, children and headteachers were devised in such a way as to take in the meaning of events for people, as well as what actually happened.

A good deal of previous research has been concerned with giftedness *per se* in children and with how it can be identified and developed, but without regard to its meaningfulness for the people concerned. Yet attitudes and consequent actions about giftedness can only be understood in terms of its significance. Several parents who discovered via the research that their children were no longer normal, but gifted, were distressed. They did not want their child either to be unusual or to have a changed idea of herself. Having a gifted child is not necessarily a happy event. Thus, a comparison of the circumstances in which some parents have sought action on behalf of their believed gifted child with those who have not was expected to throw light on the meaningfulness of the term gifted to different people.

In spite of their action, it could not be assumed before beginning the research that parents who sought help were more in need of it than others who had not. There are many reasons for such parental behaviour. Nor could children who have been nominated as gifted be supposed to represent all gifted children in the community, so that general conclusions might be drawn from them. Yet children nominated by parents and teachers have actually been considered as typical gifted children in other researches (Hitchfield, 1973; Painter, 1976).

Joining an association for gifted children supposes several underlying psychological decisions. The first is one of the acceptability of the image. To announce that one has a gifted child is, in an essentially 'protestant' society, an immodest claim – although it is better than announcing an unruly, unhappy child. However, the combination of the two in the current mythology that giftedness equals problems is perfectly acceptable.

The second decision is one of motivation, which is influenced both by the social environment and by personality factors. It is not only a matter of personal choice, but also of cultural expectation as to how and when one seeks contact with an outside agency. Some people are expected within their culture to keep their troubles to themselves, while others feel free to call for assistance without much hesitation. But even within the same culture, some people react to the same adversity by soldiering on, where others would give up.

In any particular problem, there are various different causes which will have been significant in its formation. These provoking agents can be inborn or be the products of life events. It is possible that the parents' action of seeking help would have come about in any case, but was triggered off by their belief in their child's giftedness.

The provoking agents for the NAGC parents were their children's unhappiness, difficult behaviour or poor performance at school. The presence, type and frequency of these problems was fairly evenly spread along the 60 IQ points range of the target children. There were also secondary provoking agents which determined the direction in which the parents turned in seeking help. These were socio-economic class influences and the parents' – particularly the mothers' – ambitions for their children. Judging by the social class membership of the NAGC the same provoking agents, if acting upon lower-class parents, would make them seek help in other directions, if at all.

Some parents would be more vulnerable than others and so would be more likely to seek outside help: for instance, those of unusual family circumstances or individual families isolated from supportive relatives and friends. Possibly some children themselves are innately more vulnerable to life events than other children and so are found to be more difficult to manage. There must be a point at which vulnerability reaches such a level that the advent of the provoking agent brings about either action or another form of collapse. The latter would be taken up by other, non-voluntary helping agencies.

The covert reasons why people join together for a common cause are at least as important as the overt ones. Parent members of the NAGC can join whether their children are gifted or not – and some of them were not. But there is an assumption in joining that some extra attention will be given to the children because of their presumed gifts. It was often explained to me by parents in the association that their children only behaved badly because they were gifted. Therefore, it was important to know whether the children's behaviour was due to parental expectation (or hope) or to other causes. In fact, many gifted children who were discovered in the process of the research had not been recognized as such by their parents, were not seen as problems and were doing well at school.

This research was carried out in such a way that the children and their environments could be looked at from many angles. When the parents who had joined the NAGC were compared with those who had not, some highly significant differences were seen between them. The NAGC mothers were particularly intriguing as having had a far better education and occupying a higher occupational status than the control mothers, but still they were less satisfied with what they had received.

Although they led a lively and cultured life, they were more likely to be left with the responsibility for their child's educational welfare. In this review of research on gifted children, Vernon found that 'The children of over-anxious mothers tend to be above average in verbal ability' (1957, p. 66). This also appeared to be true for the children and their mothers in this present study.

Fathers of the target children had a similar outlook on life to that of the mothers, though to a lesser extent. But their relatively smaller involvement with the children could have been detrimental. Other research work has found that the active involvement of the father in the child's life seemed an essential ingredient for effective adaptation at home and at school (Love and Kaswan, 1974; Pilling and Kellmer Pringle, 1978). The children of the one-parent families in the sample, who only had mothers, were showing signs of that deprivation. The target group parents of both sexes had been very successful in their own careers and had high expectations of their children's future success. They also put notably more achievement pressure on their children than other parents.

When the home backgrounds were compared, on the basis of the children's measured IQs, a different picture emerged, though. The parents of children of over 140 IQ had very high levels of education and occupational status, but they lacked any element of dissatisfaction. They were particularly helpful to their children's educational progress, in respect of both provision and encouragement, and did put some pressure on them to succeed. The home backgrounds of the children of high IQ were culturally extremely active, especially in literature and music. Comparing the home backgrounds of children who had been rated along a range of adjustment, they were not found to vary significantly, except in the make-up of the immediate family. Where there had been some disturbance in the family, the child was less well adjusted.

Parents and teachers were in considerable agreement as to the development and adjustment of the children. The target children were seen by both as being troubled; parents described problems seen in the home, such as sensitivity, emotionality and poor sleep. This last is probably an aspect of social class; in general, the higher up the social ladder the parents are, the more sleep they expect of their children (Lawson and Ingleby, 1974). These particular parents in the study were, if not already high up, upwardly mobile.

The children of the target group were also described by their parents as independent, possessing excellent memories and making good school progress, in comparison with their control children. But they were also said to 'feel different' 17 times more often than the control children. These aspects of 'gifted' behaviour which the target parents described for their children were not found when the children of measured high IQ were compared with children of moderate IQ. The outstanding aspect of the development of the high IQ children was their advanced verbal ability in reading and in talking – not their emotional problems. The high IQ children were, however, independent and were said to 'feel different'. They had extraordinary memories, could concentrate for great lengths of time, and were lively and active in their leisure pursuits, but did not have many friends. Their handwriting was poor. The children of the sample who were poorly adjusted were also seen by their parents as 'feeling different' across the whole sample range of IQ. But they were also seen as 'difficult' and were faring badly at school. They too had poor handwriting.

The most dramatic and telling discoveries in the project were those of the teachers' descriptions of the children's adjustment in the classroom, which was assessed by their overt behaviour. Target children were seen as very much less well adjusted than either of the control groups, at a high level of statistical significance. Teachers found the target children to be disturbed nearly twice as often as the control children. Parents' decisions to join the association for gifted children were clearly related to the children's behaviour.

There was always the possibility that the distress shown by the target group children was due to the educational frustration of the gifted amongst them attending a non-specialist school. Therefore, the whole sample was compared for adjustment in terms of their IQ scores. Teachers' reports of the children's adjustment behaviour in school showed that there was absolutely no difference between the High and Moderate IQ groups. It was apparent that there were no differences in children's school behaviour that were due to IQ alone; the behaviour of the target children must have been due to other reasons. This poor adjustment within the target group was spread fairly evenly across their IQ range. But the target group contained all the sample children who combined poor adjustment with a high IQ and about half of them were failing at school. These undoubtedly gifted but unhappy children whose parents had joined the association were not found to represent other gifted non-members. The precipitating factor which moved these parents to action appeared to be the children's behaviour, along with a fairly high IQ.

# DEVELOPMENTAL EVIDENCE OF GIFTEDNESS

## Early development

## Alertness at birth

It was only the target children who were described as more alert at birth, in comparison with the control groups. This is a feature of children which has been mentioned as an early indication of their giftedness by Gesell (1950) and others. However, there were no differences in reported early alertness between the high IQ children and the moderate IQ children, nor between the adjustment groups.

It cannot be said therefore, on the evidence from this study, that children who are intellectually gifted are objectively more alert at birth. It is possible that a high proportion of the target parents were anticipating a very bright child, even before the baby's birth, and readily accepted their own and the nurses' descriptions of their babies as 'bright' or 'clever' in support of this. No one has ever investigated how often newborn babies are complimented in this way, but this present research may have provided some evidence as to how seriously such remarks may be taken by some parents.

## Walking

Most children can be expected to be walking well and independently by 15-18 months (Gessell, 1950; Davie *et al.*, 1972; Tanner, 1978). But Terman (1925) found that his sample of gifted children were walking, on average, one month earlier than the norm. However, as Tanner points out, social class difference affect the age by which children pass their developmental milestones.

In this sample, the target children were described as walking significantly earlier than their controls. But it was very surprising to find that the high IQ children were not described as walking earlier than the moderate IQ children. When social class is held relatively constant, as it was in this sample, the physical developmental milestone of walking did not emerge as being directly related to measured IQ. There is a strong possibility that in other studies, where gifted children were found to walk earlier than other children, their generally superior home backgrounds, which have enabled the children to score highly on the IQ test and helped their superior physical status, have also provided the reason for their early walking. In this sample, though, intellectual giftedness was not found to be related to early walking.

## Talking

Infants can be expected to be using one or two words other than 'mama' or 'dada' at 12 months, and by 24 months should be speaking in short sentences (Gessell, 1950; Davie *et al.*, 1972). Girls may be rather more advanced than boys in this respect, but there do not seem to be clear social class effects on talking at this early stage. Bridges (1973), among others, has pointed out that many gifted children learn to speak earlier than their contemporaries, speak fluently and have good sentence structure and a wide vocabulary. Indeed, Terman found that his gifted sample talked on average $3\frac{1}{2}$ months earlier than the norm.

In my sample, the target children were described by their parents as talking early twice as frequently as either of the control groups. When the children were regrouped and compared in terms of IQ, the high IQ children were again described as talking early twice as often as the moderate IQ children. There were no differences in this respect between the adjustment groups. It is concluded from this research that intellectually gifted children do talk much earlier than normal children.

## Reading

Research results on the question of when gifted children begin to read are confused and much of the work which has been carried out into it is American. This makes comparison with Britain difficult, as most reading skills are acquired in schools and British children start school in their fifth year, while American children start when they are six years old. Although it is often said that gifted children tend to be self-taught, it might be expected that some adult had an interpretive role in the teaching.

Social class and sex are known to affect reading attainment, favouring the higher social classes and girls. But whether or not the gifted child becomes an avid or omnivorous reader at an early age depends not only on her background, but on personality structure and mental adjustment; reading problems and maladjustment are closely linked. Some gifted children seem to read in a very selective manner, using books for reference when a specific piece of information is sought (Tempest, 1974).

An unexpected finding in this sample was that the target children started reading later than the control-one group, who had been matched for intelligence. They had walked and talked earlier, but read later; they were also very much less well adjusted. Although they included many intellectually gifted children, their early reading skills were at a level very little above those of randomly selected schoolmates (the control-two group).

The high IQ children, however, presented a dramatically different picture when compared with the moderate IQ children. Their early reading skills were almost twice as frequent as those of the moderate IQ group. When compared for adjustment, those children who were badly adjusted were not found to be doing well in any scholastic endeavour. Intellectually gifted children thus appeared to be prominent in their verbal precocity, both in talking and reading. The validity of high verbal achievement as an indication of intellectual giftedness is greatly strengthened by this evidence.

As they grew older, the children who had been so verbally precocious became much more avid and wider readers than is usual. The intellectually gifted children were described as having a broad span of reading and the children confirmed this in their self-descriptions. The target children too, when compared to their controls, were said by their parents to read more, but the target children in their self-descriptions did not seem to be particularly keen on reading as a pastime.

## General Development

### Sleep

Most lists of characteristics by which a gifted child might be identified contain a reference to the generally accepted idea that the gifted child needs less sleep than other children. Perhaps the main reason for the confusion over this aspect of child behaviour is that investigators ask parents and not children whether a sleep problem exists. The estimation of a 'problem' in turn depends on the parents' ideas of what constitutes difficulty in sleep.

In their study referred to earlier, Lawson and Ingleby (1974) found that what was considered to be 'normal' sleeping time for a child varied by a difference of hours between families. In general, the higher the social class of the family, the longer the child was expected to sleep. Additionally, if the parental role is played in a relatively permissive way, then the child may be allowed to amuse herself with books and toys during her time in bed and it is unlikely that a 'problem' will arise. If the parents see their role in a more authoritarian light, then the child may be required to lay still, stop reading, be quiet, etc. If this routine is carried out before the child is ready for sleep, then a 'problem' is very likely to develop.

When asked about their children's sleeping habits, half the parents of the target children said their children had sleep problems; this was many times more than the control children. The target children were also said to sleep very much less than the control children. When the high IQ children were compared with children of moderate ability, although the differences in sleep patterns were not significant, the high IQ children did seem to sleep less well. But if the sleep patterns of the high and moderate IQ children were compared without the target children, the high IQ children were then seen to sleep at least as soundly as the moderate IQ children. It was decidedly the target children who had the sleep problems.

In the comparison between the adjustment groups for sleep problems, surprisingly there had been no significant differences between the groups. However, by scrutinizing the parents' remarks, additional to their answers to the questionnaire, it was found that they did complain more about the sleep of the less well adjusted children. Of all the children described as having poor sleep, over two-thirds were target children. In fact, from every angle of enquiry, it was the children of parents who had joined the NAGC who appeared to be the ones with 'sleep problems'.

## Physical health

The children's physical health, as described by both parents and teachers, was found to differ for the various groups. That of the target group was particularly poor when compared to the control groups; these children were described as having very unsatisfactory co-ordination and many respiratory/nervous complaints. Apart from their poorer eyesight, the list of physical complaints from which they suffered is indicative of the presence of anxiety. When the children of high and moderate IQ respectively were compared, without the target children, no differences were found in physical health, but the children who were poorly adjusted were found to be less physically fit than the better adjusted ones. The relationship between physical and mental health is discussed on p. 77.

## Physical stature

Although the popular stereotype of the gifted child is that of a weak, bespectacled 'weed', much research has shown that this is not true (Terman, 1925; Tempest, 1974; Ogilvie, 1973). But it must be noted that factors such as social class, birth order, parents' height, child's birth weight and early nourishment all affect physical stature (Davie *et al.*, 1972; Tanner, 1978). Children of professional parents are physically superior to others and score more highly on tests of mental ability than smaller or less mature children. These effects may be environmental or genetic, or probably the interaction of both. We are thus faced with the question: are these children taller because they are gifted, or gifted because they are taller, and are both these effects a by-product of their parents' socio-economic level?

This research has been particularly useful in throwing some light on the question of environment. The social class of the parents of the whole sample was relatively homogeneous; they were mostly of high social class and well educated. None of the sample could be described as poor, though there was a tiny minority of upwardly aspiring working class families. As the research project did not have the means to examine the children medically, all the physical descriptions of the children were given by their school teachers on the form (BSAG) which they completed. This had the advantage that they were able to compare each child in question with the rest of her classmates. Contrary to others' findings, the teachers did not describe the gifted children as taller than their classmates in this sample. The reason is probably that without the influence of the home background factor, IQ of itself does not affect the height of children.

## Eyesight

The target children in my research were described twice as often as the control children as having poor eyesight. Yet when the total sample was examined in terms of IQ scores, the children of high IQ were found to have equally good eyesight as those of moderate IQ. When the children of high and moderate IQ were compared without the target children, those of high IQ were found to have somewhat better eyesight than those of moderate IQ. It seemed as though there was a particularly high rate of poor eyesight in the target group, which was not so for the other groups, and there were no differences between the adjustment groups with regard to eyesight. It was unlikely, even if the target group children were suffering from more anxiety than the others, that it would affect their vision.

Intellectual attainment and short-sightedness have been linked together, both in the popular stereotype of the gifted child and also in the results of research. Observations on 3775 children of the National Survey Sample Cohort by Douglas and his team revealed a link between short-sightedness and intellectual attainment (Douglas, 1964 and 1968). They found that short-sighted children, compared with those of good vision, were hard working, more attentive in class and had more academic hobbies. They also did better at school because of the extra encouragement and support they received from home. Parents of short-sighted children were more likely to be interested in their children's education and progress at school than parents of children with normal sight. The team related the children's eyesight to achievement at school, family background, the parents' own education and attitudes to their children's education. All the children in the cohort had their eyes tested and they were also given intelligence tests (verbal, non-verbal and mathematical). No relationship was found between intelligence and short-sightness.

In his study of gifted children who were chosen on the basis of their high achievement, Terman (1925) also found a high incidence of defective vision, although his group were above average on most health measures. This strange state of affairs has not as yet been explained. It is possible that when children have to peer more closely at their books, the side-effect is an increase in concentration. This seemingly greater effort on the part of the children to learn would positively reinforce the parents to greater encouragement. A positive cycle is then set up whereby children and parents (as well as teachers) reinforce each other to produce the best school results of which the child is capable. The alternative situation could equally well arise, however, that children who find it difficult to see could become discouraged by the extra effort required to read and give up more readily. But all the available evidence indicates that this alternative is not the usual reaction of short-sighted children.

The idea of the positive cycle of school achievement probably holds true for short-sighted children, as it does for other children who show an apparently positive inclination for school work. But seen in the general medical and social context short-sightedness, like other dysfunctions, is observable as part of a wider constellation of problems. Such seemingly innocuous conditions as irregular teeth and poor hearing are known to occur along with other quite different disorders and children who visit doctors for any reason are statistically more likely to have more physical problems in general than those who do not. An example of this constellation of symptoms is found in children who are accident-prone. Children who are seen by paediatric surgeons because of the consequences of a seemingly pure accident have been found to have many more general health and emotional troubles than children who are not the victims of accidents.

Even though the numbers in my sample of children are not large, they provide statistically significant results. The children who had poor eyesight were far more likely to have other physical problems, but they also came from educationally supportive homes and were achieving well at school. It is my contention that, had these been measured, they would also have shown more problems such as orthodontic or hearing irregularities. Similarly, American orthodontists might well find that children who wore dental braces did better at school than those who did not, but such a survey would be worthless in Britain, where the sight of a child's teeth contained by metal is unusual.

## Curiosity and interests

Both parents and teachers see great curiosity as an indication of giftedness (Tempest, 1974; Shields, 1968; Ogilvie, 1973), though it is not the quantity of questions which distinguish the gifted child but their quality. Questions may be showered on parents as a means of disrupting other activities or of attracting attention. There is the possibility that teachers may see as gifted questioners only those children who ask the 'right' kind of questions, i.e. those which fit into the teacher's own mental framework. In fact, social class differences were reported when teachers were asked to assess their pupils' awareness of the world around them (Davie, Butler and Goldstein, 1972). The children in my sample had a similar social class background, but the teachers were not found to discriminate between them in general terms of attractiveness, no matter how they were grouped.

The parents in this sample, when asked to describe their gifted children, were not specific about the children's curiosity. However, when the children were asked about themselves and the high IQ children were compared with those of moderate IQ they were seen as having significantly wider, livelier and more cultural (especially musical) interests. The target children, when compared with the controls, were not found to have significantly wider interests, but they did play more music. The conclusion which may be drawn from this and more general supporting information is that gifted children are indeed more curious than normal children. Not only that, but they follow it up with enthusiasm as far as they are able.

Children of very high IQ seemed to have keen powers of observation, judging by the way they pursued their interests. Their active and lively minds were not slow to appreciate beauty, which implies a fine perceptual ability. I had found in earlier research (Freeman, 1977) that aesthetic appreciation in children is considerably influenced by home backgrounds. Children who were identifiably talented in the appreciation and practice of music or fine art came from homes where such matters were held to be important. The gifted children in this present sample also came from homes where aesthetic appreciation was considered to be important and were encouraged both to practise and investigate it, to the wide extent which was possible for them.

Differences were found between the parents' and the children's descriptions of how the children occupied their time, particularly with regard to television watching. Target parents, when compared to control parents, said their children preferred the educational type of television programmes – when they watched it at all. But when the children were asked what they enjoyed on television, they gave a wide range of favourite programmes. In the comparisons between the IQ groups and the adjustment groups, the children's television watching habits were not found to be significantly different, as described by the parents. But again the children seemed to enjoy almost whatever was put before them; the favourite programmes of gifted children were no different from those of normal children. But the amount of time they spent watching television, and sometimes what they watched, was directed by the parents.

## Energy

Many writers about gifted children have commented that they have more than the normal allowance of physical and mental energy and that these children are very active and exuberant in what they do (Ogilvie, 1973; Bridges, 1973; Vernon *et al.*, 1977). There is, of course a difference between being exceptionally energetic and being over-active (or hyperactive), although even exceptional energy can cause problems both at home and school as parents and teachers become exhausted in trying to cope with it.

Over-activity may cause difficulties with concentration on school work and the child may consequently fail to make satisfactory progress there. Sex and social class differences favour the middle class girl, when teachers are asked to rate children on over-activity in the classroom (Stott, 1976). Here, behaviour norms are implicated, as with so many judgements, and of course the tolerance levels of the parents or teacher for a 'bouncy' child are also important.

Parents who joined the NAGC did not describe their children as more energetic than the controls. In fact, in terms of physical energy, the control-one group who had been matched for intelligence played far more sport than either the target group or the control-two group, who had been chosen at random. When the children were compared for their high or moderate IQ, it was the moderate IQ children who were described as livelier by their parents than were the high IQ children. However, of the children who were described by their teachers as poorly adjusted, a very high proportion were seen as being hyperactive. It was also the less well adjusted children who were not doing well at school.

This research has provided evidence to show that intellectually gifted children are indeed mentally more lively and energetic than normal children, but they cannot be described as physically more energetic. Their interests tend to be of an intellectual, cultural nature rather than sport, for instance.

## Co-ordination

Problems with poor co-ordination can result in poor handwriting and poor achievement in school. Fine motor control seems to be more difficult for boys than for girls and for lower rather than upper class children. But these differences could well be related to expected behaviour norms and social training in the different groups. Thus, when Illingworth (1964) writes that 'Advanced manipulative development in a baby is of much more importance as a sign of mental superiority than is gross mental development', he appears to disregard the effects of social conditioning.

Of the children in this sample, the target children, when compared to their controls, were described – especially by parents – as having very much poorer co-ordination. When the children were compared for IQ no differences were found in co-ordination between the groups, but there were differences between the adjustment groups. There was almost a sliding scale indicating that the less well adjusted a child, the less well co-ordinated he was found to be. Clearly, the children who were seen as troubled with poor co-ordination were those whose parents had joined the NAGC and those who were poorly adjusted. The questions asked to elicit this information were, for example: Can he ride a bicycle? Does he knock into things when he's moving about? Answers to such questions were considered to refer to gross motor activities.

Fine motor control can be seen most easily in handwriting and parents were asked whether they considered their child's handwriting to be good, bad or indifferent. No differences were described between the handwriting efficiency of the target and control groups. Remembering that the target group had been described as particularly poor in co-ordination, it might have been expected that their handwriting would reflect this, but it did not. However, when the children were compared for IQ, the high IQ children had very much poorer handwriting than those of moderate IQ. The adjustment groups again seemed to have a sliding scale of handwriting, viz. the poorer the child's adjustment, the less good her handwriting.

In this research, then, the two categories of highly intelligent and poorly adjusted children were found to have poor handwriting, but it is suggested that there were different causes behind the standard of writing of each group. The poorly adjusted children were in general doing badly at school and were a problem to their parents at home. Although some of them were highly intelligent, their personal problems seemed to get in the way of application and effectiveness in their lives. Their handwriting was but one aspect of this. The high IQ gifted children, who were achieving well in almost every direction, were another matter. They were probably impatient of 'reproductive communication' and found writing too slow for their thought processes. The high IQ children were the only group that had said of themselves that 'sometimes the world was too slow' for them. Their bad handwriting, especially in the early years of school, could allow the teacher to under-estimate gifted children's ability.

# Memory

Many researchers have found that the gifted child has an exceptionally good memory from a very early age and brings it into play when gathering his store of general knowledge. Teachers, however, do not seem to regard good memory as a reliable indication of giftedness (Ogilvie, 1973).

The parents of the target group reported twice as often as the control parents that their children had extraordinarily good memories. Parents of the high IQ children mentioned this feature two and a half times more often than parents of the moderate IQ group. Memory does not seem to be affected by the level of a child's adjustment and it may reasonably be considered that the possession of an exceptional memory is a distinct sign of intellectual giftedness.

# Concentration

A high level of concentration is often described as a feature of gifted children and, clearly, the ability to concentrate can assist achievement in any endeavour. In comparison with their controls, the target children's parents did not see their children as having significantly greater powers of concentration. However, when the children were compared on the basis of IQ, the picture changed dramatically; the parents of the high IQ children described them as able to concentrate for many hours nearly three times as often as the parents of the moderate IQ children. Not surprisingly, of these high IQ children, over half were described as making excellent school progress. This ability to concentrate deeply and for great lengths of time is certainly a feature of the intellectually gifted child.

# Understanding

It is likely that the gifted child may show the logical powers of an older child. She may also have a great ability to see relationships between objects and ideas and to apply them in new situations. It could be expected that the gifted child would be advanced in her levels of intellectual development; she may even jump whole stages in an argument or logical progression, though unable to describe how she reached the answer. This can be disconcerting to teachers. She may also see ambiguities in questions which others do not see, causing her to pause and consider before answering and thus appearing to be slow in response.

This research was not concerned with the finer details of cognitive growth in gifted children. An attempt was made, though, to discover how the children saw life and their place in their own environment. But possibly, due to the inherent conformity of children of the age of this sample, they seemed to be loathe to make firm statements about their feelings. A very frequent and seemingly defensive answer to many questions was 'don't know'; the alternative was 'sometimes'. However, the gifted children were found to think differently from the other children.

Both the target children (who were two-thirds gifted) when compared to their controls, and the high IQ children when compared to the moderate IQ children were more able to empathise, i.e. to see life through another's eyes. They were also able to pay attention to more than one thing at once. Such children could, for example, listen to two conversations at the same time or watch television and read a book. The children were very specific as to whether they could or could not do this; there was no hesitation in reply. It does not seem to be a facility which one has more or less of; one can either do it or one can't.

## Achievement

The question of achievement has been discussed earlier, in Chapter 3; the criteria by which it might be measured are as variable as the children's homes and schools they attended. In this research, achievement was taken as what was perceived by parents and teachers, whether that was good or bad. The teacher's judgement will be affected by the level prevailing in the school class, the parents' probably by a wide variety of reasons.

Pringle (1970) wrote that 'a high incidence of emotional difficulties' was a characteristic found among under-achieving able children. Less than half of her sample of over IQ 130 children were judged by their teachers as being of good or very good ability. She wrote that 'such a serious under-estimate suggests that teachers judge intelligence primarily by a pupil's level of achievement'. On this reasoning, a child who under-achieves yet is highly intelligent and unrecognized as such may enter a vicious circle that could lead to maladjustment. That a child might be doing badly at school and yet still have a high intelligence is an idea which many teachers and parents find difficult to credit.

232

Social class, parental attitudes to education and home stability have often been found to affect children's achievement in school. Pringle believes that the roots of under-achievement are to be found in the home during the early years of life. The child's personality, sibling relationships, emotional adjustment in the home and school all combine and interact to affect the child and his readiness and willingness to learn.

The target children in my sample, when compared to the control children, were on the whole seen by their parents as doing well at school and 43% were doing extremely well. These parents, however, were less happy about the school than the parents of the control children in the same school class. The high IQ group children, when compared to the moderate IQ group children, were described by their parents as doing well and 55% as doing extremely well. But the children compared for their school progress in terms of their adjustment rating seemed to be on a sliding scale – the worse the adjustment, the worse they did at school. Of the most poorly adjusted children, 48% were said to be doing badly at school.

When the teachers were asked to comment on the children's achievement in school, their descriptions did not differentiate between the different groupings in the sample. They did not, for example, see the gifted children as achieving better than the rest of the class. The reason for this very probably is that the teacher adjusted her idea of achievement to what the child in question seemed capable of achieving. But I too found, as Pringle did, that teachers did not spot the gifted child who was achieving at very much below the level of his potential. The children did seem to be seen in terms of what they did, rather than in terms of what they could do, even though some of them were clearly described by the teachers as maladjusted. It looks as though gifted children in the danger zone of maladjustment and under-achievement are not being recognized or assisted. Are their many physical health problems cries for help?

## Personality development

The likelihood of gifted children being recognized among the upper social class levels may be the reason why giftedness is associated with favourable personality characteristics in some researchers' eyes. Gallagher (1975) reports a study by Bonsall and Stefflre (1955) in which gifted boys were compared with youngsters of average intelligence. The gifted boys were found to be generally superior in their personality traits, including 'masculinity'. However, when the two groups were controlled for socio-economic level, virtually no differences were found between the groups. Bonsall and Stefflre concluded 'It is possible that Terman in describing the multiple superiority of the gifted child is simply describing children from the upper socio-economic levels'. If this is so, then many assumptions about the personality 'differences' of the gifted which appear to call for special educational approaches will need to be reconsidered. With these home-background influences controlled as much as is humanly possible, the following aspects of personality development in gifted children were discovered in my research.

## Adjustment

There is a danger that the maladjusted gifted child will go unrecognized in the classroom, as teachers often do not consider that a delinquent or unpopular child could be gifted. In my sample, there were two out of the 82 gifted children who were described as below average ability by their teachers. Both were maladjusted and had problems at home. In these two cases, there did not seem to be any way in which the teacher's recognition of their giftedness would have helped their maladjustment. It was perhaps better for them at that time to keep a low profile in class; this was the only tranquillity of the day. Should children such as these two grow up to be a menace to society, the root of their delinquency would not be in their giftedness, though, but in their home backgrounds or in themselves.

In her study of 'Able Misfits', Pringle (1970) found that too high or too low parental expectations often contributed to the child's maladjustment. Unhappy homes, illogical parental discipline and 'inconsistent handling' occurred more in the able misfit group than in the population as a whole. She suggested that 'good intellectual ability by itself is insufficient to compensate for inadequate parental support and interest'. Studies reported by Gallagher (1975) have all shown that gifted children, of very high IQ, are better adjusted than less able children.

Parents' attitudes towards their gifted children can range from being overly proud to denying that the child is exceptional at all. Typical comments from the parents of gifted children who did not join the NAGC were:

> Child IQ 166; 'We don't think he's outstanding. Not bright enough to be a problem'.

Child IQ 162; 'He's not outstanding; he's very happy'.

Child IQ 149; 'He's got a marvellous memory, but he's very affectionate'.

The old stereotype of 'giftedness equals unhappiness' seems to have influenced these parents into being unaware of their children's unusually high abilities. Many also said that their child was clever, but 'normal'. As a researcher who knew of the children's rare ability, I found that parents did not always want to share this information, nor could I see where it would necessarily have benefited the child. Those who wanted to know and were told often described their feelings of fear: 'I didn't know – but we were so happy – he's happy. Should I have guessed? What shall I do? I'm frightened'. Problems of adjustment have been discussed earlier in Chapter 3.

The target children in this sample were outstandingly less well adjusted as described by their teachers, when compared with their controls. Some suffered from symptoms of withdrawal, but most overreacted, acting without thinking, were generally hostile and found it difficult to make friends. Parents described these target children as emotional, poor sleepers, particularly sensitive and difficult to bring up. The teachers and parents appeared to be in close agreement as to who the ill-adjusted children were.

However, when the children were compared on their IQ scores for the same items, there were no significant differences in those adjustment behaviours between the high and moderate IQ children. It has been shown many times in this research that high IQ in a child does not bring about unhappiness or bad behaviour of itself.

The distinguishing behavioural features of the poorly adjusted children at school were the same as those of the target group. But parental complaints were more evenly spread over the three levels of adjustment that were compared. The one feature of which there was no doubt was that the child concerned was 'difficult' at home and a problem in the classroom. He was likely to be a boy, to be gifted and to have unusual home circumstances.

It cannot be said, though, that intellectual giftedness and maladjustment are directly related. Whatever reasons brought about the various levels of maladjustment of the children in this sample would be expected to produce the same results in children of all levels of ability. However, the combination of giftedness and maladjustment is potentially powerful in the damage it can do to society. Of the 210 children of above average ability in this sample, only ten came into this category, i.e. 2.1%. The proportion in the general population must be about 1%, but even so, that is a lot of potentially dangerous children who have at present very little recognition or help. In Britain, it is only the National Association for Gifted Children which offers help, but it depends on voluntary assistance, especially out of London, and simply has not the means to help all the difficult gifted children in the country.

## Independence

The abilities to work alone and with self-confidence are often seen as facets of the gifted child's personality. This is, of course, also affected by opportunity and parental attitudes. The budding film director needs more than ideas to practice with. Pringle (1970) found that among her 'able misfits' group, few children were given above average opportunities for gaining independence. More boys than girls were given such opportunities and more children in non-manual homes than in professional, managerial or manual homes.

The target children in my sample were described by their parents as significantly more independent than the two control groups. So too were the high IQ group, when compared with the moderate IQ group. But the independence of the high IQ gifted children seemed to extend into other aspects of their lives; their interests were particularly wide and varied. They seemed to be able to stand back and see things more objectively than children of less ability. For example, the gifted children were significantly less affected by the personality of their teacher than the less able children; if teachers see gifted children as a threat, perhaps this is why. The gifted child is so independent that he will go on learning, whatever the teacher sees fit to do – whether it is to appeal to the class's sense of honour, to treat them to ill-temper, to use sarcasm or make them laugh. It could be very unnerving to a teacher. The target children, although they had a high proportion of gifted children in their number, did not seem to have this great independence, but they did have a high level of poor adjustment. It is probable that they were less secure and, being so, were more dependent on adult approval and less able to be objective about their relationships with others.

The gifted children were also objectively critical about their teachers. They recognized good and bad teaching, but were also able to give teachers advice as to where they went wrong and how they could do better. They were concerned about the administration of the school and often saw their own class teacher as a fly in the spider's net of the school. Children can feel sorry for their teachers, but gifted children can suggest ways out for them. Where the teacher is attempting to hold on to her 'authoritarian' role and to put the child into a 'pupil' role, the gifted child will not fit into the scenario and will be seen as awkward. But at no point in this research did teachers describe gifted children as more difficult to teach than other children.

## Feeling different

The gifted child as she gets older probably begins to realise that she is different in some ways from other children. Hitchfield (1973) found that more of her IQ 130+ group saw themselves as 'self assertive' and 'intelligent' than did those in the under IQ 130 group. These differences could, however, have been influenced by the social class of the children in Hitchfield's series, because of her method of sampling.

This one question, asked of the parents in my sample, proved to be the most discriminating of all the 217 variables: 'Do you think your child feels different to other children?' It discriminated to a highly significant level between the three major comparisons. The target children were described as feeling very different in comparison with their controls – 50% of them were thus described; the high IQ children were described in this way in comparison with the moderate IQ children – 35% of them; and the poorly adjusted children in comparison with the better adjusted children – 52% of them.

The children whose parents described them as feeling different from other children had reason for doing so. Gifted children made up two-thirds of the target group, which also showed a high incidence of poor adjustment, at school and at home. It would perhaps have been surprising if they had not felt themselves to be different. But the high IQ group, of whom all could be said to be gifted and who were no better or worse adjusted than the moderate ability children, also felt very different. The reasons for this feeling, described by the parents regardless of whether they were members of NAGC or not, are most probably related to the very high level of their ability. Their independence, high verbal ability and wide ranging minds, bubbling with ideas, would very soon in their school lives make them aware that they were not like most of the children in the class. But, it is important to note, they did not appear to be disturbed at all by this difference. They were all happy at school, if at times objectively critical of the way it was run.

# Friends

Although there has been little factual evidence so far that gifted children prefer friends older than themselves, this has frequently been described in literature about gifted children. The evidence which I have presented here has corroborated this belief.

The target children were described by their parents, in comparison with the controls, as being without many friends. This pattern was repeated for the high IQ children, when compared with the moderate IQ children. It can be said from these results that gifted children do indeed have fewer friends than other children, and those that they do have tend to be older. Some gifted children have no friends at all, though this does not seem to trouble them.

# Self-concept

In spite of the various less-than-flattering descriptions which adults gave of the children, the children's responses to their own questions about themselves were less discriminating; none of the children actually described themselves as feeling different. They could see good and bad points about themselves, but it seemed to be of matters which are general to all children. For example, one child said that others did not like him because he did impressions of them and another said that the other girls in the road did not like her because she went to a 'posh' school. Some felt liked because they shared their sweets or had 'nice hair'. Most gifted children recognized that they were clever, but they did not see their gifts as adults do – in terms of value to society, or to their parents or to themselves. The impression received from the children's replies to questions was that they positively did not want to be seen as different, in spite of any evidence to the contrary.

## False leads

There were a number of aspects of giftedness in children which are often quoted in educational literature and which were followed-up in this research, but which produced either unclear or negative results. Some of these ideas, together with what was found, are presented below for the benefit of future researchers attempting to identify gifted children.

## Pattern of play

The evidence, acquired from nearly 6000 sets of correspondence with the NAGC, seemed to indicate that gifted children might have a developmental pattern of play or interests. The child would begin with an initial investigation of the construction of the cot, move swiftly through baby tactile exploration, lingering only with the more exciting sensations. In childhood, there seemed to be an early interest in jig-saw puzzles carried to great complicated lengths. This would be followed by interest in prehistoric animals, dinosaurs in particular. Boys then went on to trains and stamp collecting; girls went on to art work of a practical nature. Collections of all sorts seemed to be a special feature of the gifted child's interests.

In the process of the research, every interest of every child was recorded. They were rated and analysed in a variety of ways, but were not found to be as expected. There was, in fact, no identifiable pattern of play or interests which gifted children enjoyed more than other children, matched for social class, age and sex.

## Birth

There was the possibility that as older mothers are likely to have mentally sub-normal children, they could be more likely to have super-normal children. From investigation of the early correspondence, it did seem that the mothers who wrote to the NAGC were older at their child's birth than the national average. However, when the gifted children in the research were matched for age, ability, sex and school class and their mothers' and fathers' ages were examined, no differences between the ages of the gifted children's parents and the other children's parents were found. Mothers of the NAGC group were older than the national average, but so were the matched children's mothers. The reason is to be found in the educational and social status level of the mothers. A high proportion of them had had tertiary education and had not begun their families until their education had finished. The average age of mothers at the birth of the child in the research sample was 28 years.

All the mothers were asked details of the child's birth with respect to whether or not it was normal. If it was not, they were asked to say in what way. There were no differences found in this sample between gifted and non-gifted children as to the manner of their delivery.

## Sense of humour

Gifted children have often been described as having a particularly witty sense of humour. They are supposed to see and emphasise absurdities in everyday situations, to enjoy playing with words and making up nonsense words, limericks and so on. When a child is said to have a good sense of humour, he is often found to be creatively gifted (Torrance, 1962; Getzels and Jackson, 1962).

In this research, neither parents nor children gave any identifiable reasons for believing that this is so. In fact, the gifted children in this sample appeared to be particularly serious. It is possible that one of the reasons for the difference in findings is between American and English children. When Hassan and Butcher (1966) replicated in Scotland Getzels and Jackson's study of creativity, they found, as I did, that a sense of humour was not a feature of gifted children. The gifted children in my study were creative, judged by what they did, but they were not playful or particularly funny; on balance, they took life seriously.

## Sensitivity

The greater awareness and sensitivity of their children was frequently mentioned by parents in the thousands of sets of correspondence which they wrote to the NAGC. They said that their young children were often troubled by the implications of the news they see and hear on television and radio, showing concern and understanding beyond their years. The parents of the target group, which was a sub-sample of the NAGC population, did describe their children as particularly sensitive and emotional, at a high level of significance. But when the children of high IQ were compared with those of moderate IQ, they were not seen to be more sensitive or emotional on the basis of IQ alone. The target children may well have been more sensitive and emotional than other children, but they were not found to be typical of all gifted children. In this sample, the reverse seemed to be true – that gifted children took a relatively objective, non-involved view of life.

# Boredom

An aspect of giftedness which is much written and talked about is that if a child is not stretched enough at school, he may become bored and either protest at having to attend any more or, as Tempest (1974) said, 'Look round for more challenging problems and become a ringleader in all sorts of mischevious problems'. Hitchfield (1973) found that among a group of children with IQs of over 130, there was a sex difference in the reasons given for being bored at school. The boys tended to be bored because they were having to repeat work which they had already mastered, whereas the girls reported boredom in situations where they did not understand the subject being taught. This last seems to be a strange reason for highly able children to be bored and it looks as though there may be children who refuse to be 'stretched'.

While the blame for boredom is often placed upon the school, the role of parents must also be considered. For example, if the parents have a low opinion of a particular school and its teachers, this attitude towards the child's day-time environment is likely to be passed on to the child. It could make him feel bored at school even before he gets there – in a sense to please his parents. The situation will obviously be worse if parents are attempting to move the child to another school. Nevertheless, a rigid curriculum is recognized as a harbinger of boredom in many children.

Very few (less than six) of the parents in my whole sample complained of their children's boredom at school. Most of the complaints about the schools were rather vague, such as 'we're not satisfied', 'they don't stretch him enough' or 'he's getting a raw deal from the system'. Perhaps it is a compliment to the schools of North-West England that the gifted children who went to them were not more bored than other children; certainly no child said so. The dissatisfaction with the schools came from the parents and, gifted or not, the children in this sample were happy at school.

## Conclusions

The research presented in this book has dispelled some myths about the consequences of being a gifted child.

(1)    The children who were presented by their parents as 'gifted' were found to be different from their intellectual peers. They were more difficult to bring up and less well adjusted in their behaviour in school.

(2)    Parents, especially mothers, who had presented their children as 'gifted' had achieved more success in their own activities and expected more from their children than other parents.

(3)    Children presented as 'gifted' had more personal and environmental problems than their peers.

(4)    Parents who presented their child as gifted were less happy about the school than the parents of the equally able classmates.

(5)    Intellectually gifted children (measured) in non-special English education did not suffer emotionally, scholastically or physically.

(6)    Measured intellectual giftedness is not itself a cause of distress to children or parents.

The children of measured intellectual giftedness were found to be different from children of moderate ability.

(1)    They were the recipients of early, continuous stimulation and encouragement at home.

(2)    Their early verbal precocity in talking and reading was retained later.

(3)    In character, the gifted children were described as feeling 'different', but were independent, with fewer and older friends than other children.

(4)    Their very high level of intellectual ability was seen in their extraordinarily good memories, feats of concentration, lively creative activities and excellent school progress. They were quick to comprehend and to react to other people and were able to pay attention to more than one thing at once.

(5)    Their handwriting was poor.

(6)    They expected a high level of future occupation.

These marks of distinction are not problems. Where problems did exist for gifted children, they seemed to be brought about by circumstances which would adversely affect any child, or by lack of understanding from the adults who looked after them. Petty school rules were often problems, such as a five year old gifted reader obliged to keep pace with the rest of the class or barred from using the older children's library. Gifted children suffered from teacher disbelief in their abilities and so sometimes appeared to be dishonest and devious. When adults did accept the children's level of ability, it sometimes seemed to elicit some fear or uncertainty in them as to what was appropriate behaviour. Uncertain and wavering behaviour in adults is known to promote anxiety in children.

The evidence outlined above does not support the idea that gifted children should be segregated for their own good from normal children over appreciable lengths of time. The minority of gifted children who did have problems were also found to have a cluster of disturbing environmental influences. The great majority of gifted children co-existed happily and prosperously alongside children of moderate ability. Fortunately for those gifted children who need it, an association now exists to help them, but whether a more 'stretching' education would improve their happiness is doubtful. Both Terman (1925) and myself, separated by 6000 miles and 50 years, have found gifted children to be emotionally and physically at least as sound as other children. We also agree that their development and future success in life is very dependent on their social environments.

# GROWING UP GIFTED

Many gifted children and their families became known to me during the course of the research and some will now be described.

The parents of children believed to be gifted not only referred to their children as sensitive and emotional, but often appeared to be so themselves. Some seemed to see themselves and, by extension, their children as victims of a system which they might fight, but had little control over. Several parents explained to me that if only they had more money they could get their child out of the state system and buy him an expensive private education, which they believed would have been better for a gifted child. Over half the parents had in fact done this, but many of them were still dissatisfied. The mother of a gifted seven year old at a private school with an entrance examination complained that 'he is held back with the dim children'. This boy, Bennie, was an only child; he had two rooms in the house for himself and his playroom was immaculate, as was his bedroom. He played chess with his father most nights and had a chess tutor once a week. He also had a language lesson, a violin lesson and a swimming lesson each week, all of them requiring practice. The behaviour of this only son was so 'terrible' and occupied so much of the parents' time that they said they could not consider having any more children. His parents had applied to join the NAGC in his first year, but the Association refused to accept him until he was four. I last saw this 'terrible' seven year old being taken, unprotesting, to the first day of the sales in a large department store; his problem behaviour was clearly only related to expectations.

Another young gifted boy was having difficulties with his father, a strict Scots disciplinarian, who believed firmly in corporal punishment at school. There was an obvious strain in the home between the boy, his mother and his domineering father. Neither of the parents liked the boy's school, in spite of its expense. Not surprisingly, the boy was showing problems in behaviour.

A brilliant little girl of five years was having problems getting dressed after the gymnastics class at her infant school. Her parents were worried and asked me whether her outstanding fluency in ancient Hebrew was inhibiting her normal development in other ways. Her teacher was becoming impatient with her slowness and they feared that she would be slighted at school. It appeared that she had trouble tying the laces in her shoes and buttoning her dresses down the back. I suggested slip-on shoes and a buttonless jumper for the time being. They also feared for her intellect since she was progressing 'too' well in Hebrew. I could only propose ancient Greek for the requested stretching – as a half-serious suggestion. The five year old took this up enthusiastically, with a private tutor, and was blissfully happy at school when visited a year later.

The mother of a gifted six year old, Charles, was almost blind. They lived in a house on a cold windy hilltop. Father was away a lot of the time and she struggled against great odds to mind her child, cook and do housework. Unfortunately, the little boy was very mischievous, given to such dreadful acts as flicking up little girls skirts and running away. The neighbours complained and the mother worried so much that she took him to the doctor. There, she was told that this was the result of her over-stimulating her son so that his brain was over-developed. The school was of the same opinion. There are obviously some people who believe that too many nursery rhymes can harm your health. She joined the NAGC, who arranged for the boy's IQ to be tested; they were pleased to accept Charles and were ready to help in any way, but because of her domestic circumstances, she could not join in any activities and the school saw this act of joining the association as offensive to them. The boy's giftedness was certainly not a blessing at that time.

Veronica's mother explained how rude and obstinate her eight year old was; she did not know of her daughter's giftedness. As an example of rudeness, her mother said that when they were out walking and she asked the younger children the names of flowers, Veronica would always jump in with the correct answer. Consequently, she was obliged to tell her little 'know-all' to be quiet when the younger children were around. Mother put it down to the fact that Veronica had 'big-sister' ideas above her station. In this case, the only son of average ability was scheduled for expensive boarding school education while Veronica was to continue in the tiny convent school. I had the impression that knowing of Veronica's giftedness would ease the tension in the house so that she might be allowed to develop in her own way.

Nine year old George's parents were recently divorced and his father had joined the NAGC on his behalf. This father was a very dominant man who had impressed the headmaster of the school with his own intellectual superiority. When George transferred to another school during the research, the headmaster said that he'd lost the finest pupil the school had ever had and refused to continue with the research because George's father was no longer involved. Fortunately, I already had the agreement of the two control families. George lived with his mother in a dirty dilapidated house during the week and went to his father at weekends. He was an introverted child who did not mix well with other children, had no close friends at all, and could not keep himself occupied. His teachers thought he was deaf at first and had him tested, but found that his hearing was normal. The boy's unhappiness appeared to arise directly from his confused home circumstances. He was not achieving and could never achieve anywhere near his potential until this situation improved.

A mother who refused to participate in the research wrote that she was sure to be condemned before it started. She 'knew' that she would be branded as an incompetent mother. Her little girl had been classified as gifted by an educational psychologist, but was a very gregarious child in spite of this. In the same letter, she wrote 'but she is a "loner" at school to such an extent that we have recently changed schools to avoid disastrous mental scarring. No amount of love is ever going to make my daughter tone down her intellectual conversation so that she is thoroughly understood by her normal age range'. The stereotype of the gifted child seemed to be very strong in that household.

Parents of an undeniably gifted son, when they heard of the research, also wrote to give a very different picture. 'To ensure his normal development as a sociable little boy, we felt it necessary to explain to him that his abilities were gifts he was born with, gifts of which he was the fortunate receiver and that problems he could solve easily and quickly meant much hard work for others'. Gratitude was required, boasting was unacceptable, and encouragement of this attitude, I am sure, helped towards the establishment of his friendly and sociable nature. In late school life, he became unofficial maths coach to less gifted contemporaries and to younger boys and is now a well adjusted and responsible man.

Mary, a gifted seven year old, was very happy; her mother wrote, when approached to join the research, that she had 'attended a meeting for parents of gifted children – and a more gloomy meeting cannot be imagined! Indeed, I felt I had no business being there, as my daughter appeared to have none of the qualities that made her recognisably "gifted". She is a dedicated under-achiever, a netball fanatic and bored only when she has no-one to play with. Oppressively normal in fact!' It could well be that if Mary's parents had insisted on her achieving her potential, instead of being content with her 'under-achievement', they might have found themselves parenting a 'typical' difficult gifted child.

On hearing about the research project, a father (who is a teacher) sent me a 13-page closely typed document on his gifted son, Bob. In brief, his thesis was that the boy was so gifted that no school alone could be expected to cope with him but thanks to his understanding parents, every feature of Bob's life and interests were documented 'for the sake of all gifted children'. Unfortunately, Bob is lonely and has 'nervous debility'. His parents are hoping for a grant to enable them to send this academically outstanding boy to a small expensive boarding school as he couldn't stand the other children's chatter in a normal school. Boarding school would probably be the best thing for this sad boy as it was difficult to believe that his giftedness alone had brought about this particular situation.

The most important aspect of eleven year old Frank, as described by his mother, was his hatred of religion. She said he had become very arrogant since a psychologist had told her a year ago, in front of the boy, that he was very intelligent. He has difficulty making friends and has constant problems at school. The mother was separated from her mentally ill husband – for her children's sake. She was coping with difficult Frank and another two alone. She had joined Mensa, an organization for gifted adults, on her own behalf and NAGC for Frank. When she heard that his IQ, as measured for the research, was only 151, she expressed keen disappointment.

Andrew at ten years old was blissfully happy as the oldest of four equally gifted boys in a poor family. His father was a low paid but skilled factory hand; the house was very shabby and the four boys wore torn clothes. Mother, who was pregnant with the fifth, said she felt that one should get priorities right in life. They had spent a high proportion of their income on a piano, for example. She had for two years been taking a degree in mathematics with the Open University, but was unsure how she'd keep up with the work when the fifth baby arrived. The marriage was very happy, she said; the father took the boys to football matches and other 'male' activities while she got on with her studies. She, of course, saw to their education.

In his autobiography of working class country life in the early part of this century, Spike Mays (1969) describes how his gifts brought him no comfort. He could not go to the grammar school, even though he had won a free place, as his parents could not even afford the obligatory school cap. Consequently, he set out to look for a job, but the farmer who eventually employed him for a pittance put his dismissal kindly, but bluntly:

'It's hard for you. You aint cut out for this 'owd farm-wuk. God gave you a bit of a brain. Find another job.'

## The gifted children's thoughts

All the children in the research were asked questions about their views on life, but the answers of the gifted children were particularly interesting and a selection of their replies is presented here:

## Self-description

'I work well in school, but I've got a bad temper.' *Sarah, aged 6.*

'I am good and bad and quite clever and get my work right.' *Bennie, aged 7.*

'I help my mummy and do as I'm told mostly. Sometimes I do things which I know are wrong.' *Alastair, aged 7.*

'I am half good and half bad. Slightly tall, I have got a slightly high voice, a head like bricks and quite sharp eyesight.' *Phillip, aged 7.*

'I sulk and find it hard to accept people who call me names. I get along with people and am delighted to run errands.' *Amanda, aged 8.*

'Serious, clever, slow witted, good with hands, happy, worrier, generous.' *Dennis, aged 9.*

'I've a good memory for facts. I can concentrate on things I like. I am quite modest and rather shy. Bad – grubby, clumsy, over self-conscious. I am an outsider at times.' *Lily, aged 9.*

'Teachers like me because I get high marks in tests.' *Adrian, aged 11.*

'I like to talk to adults about certain subjects and I think they enjoy talking to me.' *Stephen, aged 11.*

'Not a goody-goody, open-minded, independent, forthright.' *Mark, aged 12.*

## How others see you

'Being good and horrid.' *Sarah, aged 6.*

'I don't play their games. I don't like them.' *Jane, aged 6.*

'I'm cheerful.' *Michael, aged 7.*

'I share my sweets and toys, but they don't like me because I'm fat.' *Alistair, aged 7.*

'They like my sort of kindness and my amusing jokes, but they dislike my thing about not helping others to do work and my way of making up games that the players do not like.' *Philip, aged 7.*

'People like me because I am clever and can do most things.' *Robert, aged 7.*

'People dislike everything about me, they like – nothing.' *Peter, aged 8.*

'Some people like me because I have wild ideas.' *Julia, aged 9.*

'I am liked because I'm not aggressive or bossy, quite good natured. I am disliked because I am aloof and don't share their interests.' *Rachel, aged 9.*

'People don't like my mixed nationality.' *Peter, aged 9.*

'People say I'm so clever, I don't know why. I don't like sport. My patience wears easily.' *Douglas, aged 11.*

'They don't like my devotion to my schoolwork.' *Alison, aged 11.*

'The girls in my road don't like me because they think I go to a posh school.' *Deborah, aged 11.*

'Some adults think I am arrogant because my parents have always allowed me to express my own opinions.' *Lawrence, aged 12.*

'Sometimes I tend to be too clever and big-headed, although I usually realize when I get into a clever mood and apologize.' *Stephen, aged 12.*

## Deep thoughts

'I think about God and sometimes wonder what it would be like to be ruler of the world.' *Alistair, aged 7.*

'I think about the hungry people of Ethiopia and the state of Britain at the moment.' *David, aged 7.*

'It's hard to think. Someone is always chatting to me.' *Philip, aged 7.*

'It would be lovely to be someone else.' *Brian, aged 7.*

'I think about how God was created, if I'd been someone else, and my place in the world.' *Amanda, aged 8.*

'I sometimes think about the pound losing its value.' *Philippa, aged 9.*

'I imagine things, like what would have happened if Churchill had lived longer and continued as Prime Minister.' *Dennis, aged 9.*

'I do not believe in God as a person. I think about politics and past civilizations.' *Jane, aged 9.*

'I pray every night, because we only go to Church once a month. I often imagine what I would do if I was famous. When political people make mistakes that cause a crisis, I think how I would avoid it, and also about the money problems of everybody.' *Lois, aged 11.*

'I often think how stupid things are like the state of Britain in the Common Market.' *Anna, aged 10.*

'I wonder how thick politicians can get.' *Brian, aged 11.*

'I don't believe in God. I sometimes think I don't have a place in the world.' *Gillian, aged 11.*

'I think that the present government is making a mess and I think that people who hold such positions should have more sense and reliability.' *Diane, aged 11.*

'I think that Britain should regain her defence commitments. Nuclear,

bacteriological warfare and chemical warfare should be banned.'
*Richard, aged 11.*

'I have thought about God, but don't feel that he exists. I feel that the
troubles of this world will end when we start sharing and get rid of all
weapons except for World Peace.' *Lawrence, aged 11.*

'Although I go to church on Sunday, I am not sure if there is an after-life.
I think it cannot be possible to die and return to life in a different place. I
also wonder how time and space can go on for ever. It all seems illogical
that there is no end to microscopic things and that however small, there
is something smaller.' *John, aged 12.*

## Problems of being gifted

There is a problem which is peculiar to children recognized as gifted
which gifted children who are unrecognized do not share. This is the
moral obligation to society to fulfil their potential. The very word gift
implies that the ability, which a child possesses to a greater extent than
most other children, is not really a consistent part of the child but has
been given to him. This extra privilege bears the burden of trust which
has to be repaid at least by the fulfilment of potential, at most by
redeeming society. This responsibility thrust on young shoulders can be
too much for them to bear. The gifted child who is badly behaved and
does not fulfil his expectations is not necessarily bored or frustrated; he
may be simply refusing to accept the burden of his gifts.

Adults who take care of the child, usually his parents, live to some
extent through him. His accomplishments are available to be experienced vicariously and serve as sources of self-esteem for relevant adults. As
the normal child grows and meets new challenges, his parents can relive
with him the pleasure of conquest. Sharing the child's success in this way
increases to some degree their own sense of effectiveness, but the
vicarious living can get out of hand. Precocity in a child can be
experienced by parents as extensions of their own lost potential so that
they become identified with their child as an image of their own
achievement. A child in this position can only let his parents down if he is
less than fully successful in every endeavour. The strain on a child can
cause considerable behaviour problems, which in terms of the myth
serve to confirm the parents' stereotyped image of their child as gifted.

The idea that the child is gifted and therefore 'odd' is as likely to be
shared by the child himself as by the rest of the population. The myth of

the disturbed gifted child is in itself disturbing to the gifted. A highly intelligent, sensitive child must question his own behaviour in relation to its acceptability. A gifted child is not expected to have a normal carefree childhood. The cares of the world are placed on the child's shoulders simply by virtue of his high ability and he is made aware of his greater responsibility for the future of us all. A child is thus expected to be a small sized diplomat whose normal childish behaviour can then be seen as 'odd'. When a gifted four year old picks quarrels it is a problem; when a normal four year old does it, he is just quarrelsome.

As gifted children grow up, they will become the recipients of a greater number and variety of 'put-downs' than most children. Adults seem to gain some sort of self-esteem, which is especially valuable to them in correcting or intellectually humiliating a gifted child. To be a 'know-all' is not a flattering description and gifted children are undoubtedly a threat to an adult's often shaky feelings of self-confidence. In some adults, the only success they have ever known is in getting the right answer for teacher at school; they are certainly not going to be upstaged by a child who really understands more now than they ever will, so their extra life experience enables them to make a clever remark or to assert their authority, which allows them to feel happier for the moment. Jealousy and fear of others' abilities, which they felt as children, can be reincarnated in adults when they meet a gifted child.

Gifted children do have more independence of mind than other children; they are less able or inclined to accept adult authority on matters of which they feel they know better. There is of course a difference between independence and obstinacy, but it sometimes depends on who is doing the perceiving. The gifted child who wants to follow up the thread of his discoveries in the classroom may be seen as obstinate by his teacher for turning unwillingly to her demands for team sports. After all, it is considered to be normal for young children to want to play games and therefore those who do not must be either obstinate or odd and maybe gifted.

Intellectually gifted children seem to face philosophical problems long before they might be expected to, whereas some children never face them at all. Problems of a God, or the function of religion, or the running of the state can beset the mind of children long before their teens. They appear because of this to be 'funny' little children, though most gifted children keep their ponderings to themselves. It is difficult to find an adult who will take a six year old's considerations on government seriously, particularly as the child only has six years' worth of information to go on. Children tend to get brushed aside with well meant suggestions to leave that consideration until they are older. In working along the paths of their own thoughts alone, without the benefit of helpful guidance, gifted children reach conclusions which may be very wide of the truth – not creative deviance but mistaken conclusions. This adds to their image of oddity.

## At school

More specific problems arise when a child goes to school. The advanced reading and verbal ability of a newcomer to school creates doubt and suspicion in the minds of many otherwise excellent teachers. Children can be coached and overcultivated so that they talk like parrots in adult language. They can be taught to regard themselves as superior and thus unable to play with other children. It is quite possible that a child who appears to be gifted is not in fact so, but has the full complement of behaviours which are mythically associated with giftedness.

The reactions of many teachers to children presented to them as gifted is to disbelieve the mother. In doing so, she may close her mind to the possibility of a child's giftedness; in that case, if the mother is able to, she can 'fight' for his recognition, but if not, the child may find it easier to pass for normal. The open-minded teacher will not, however, take long to find out the genuineness of the child's position. From the teacher's point of view, some parents are seen to insist that their child is gifted in spite of evidence to the contrary and blame her for the child's 'lack' of progress. The teacher's defences, which she sets up to counter this kind of attack, may blinker her to those children who would really benefit from appropriate education for the gifted, rather than merely relief from pressure to achieve.

All of us, child or adult, like to escape from the real world from time to time. The gifted child is often described as a day-dreamer, but that very description and its associations with sleep, indicates something about the describer. It would be equally valid to say that the child is imaginative. Gifted children can escape into their imaginations more easily than other children and can also escape into written words earlier and easier. Children who can read easily and fluently sometimes find that the printed page is more interesting than teacher's or parent's spoken word. The adult involved is not pleased by this and the child is dubbed a 'bookworm', which is not normally considered to be a flattering description. Adult distaste for children's yearning for reading probably has several psychological roots, all related to an awareness of subtle forms of rejection of the adult.

Reading is a solitary activity, being read to is not. When children learn to read fluently by themselves they no longer need a helping adult. This new ability enables a child to leave the world of the here and now and live life vicariously. Some teachers feel that when a child begins to 'go it alone' in reading, she should be ready for the experience in terms of maturity. They believe that unexpurgated reading is dangerous and confusing, which is one reason why books in schools are preselected for different age-groups. Story-telling is controlled and so is not dangerous.

A child who is able to gain new insights without the benefit of an adult also runs the danger, in some teachers' eyes, of losing touch with others. Bookworms are not very sociable, but then neither are hostile children. Books as an escape can be seen as so addictive that children should only have them in prescribed quantities, like drugs. Free access to the junior library by infants can be seen as causing problems in a young child's 'natural' development. Being obliged to play with other children when the story is just getting exciting is a handicap of childhood. Schools vary in how much social behaviour they expect of their pupils and how much they will allow the children to follow their individual styles of learning.

Gifted children who are being taught by traditional formal methods may find the imposed educational structure particularly irksome. Their teachers too can find them particularly irritating. Sometimes their thoughts are stimulated by the lesson, but in a different direction to that expected by the teacher. Gifted children often feel a mild resentment at having to do what the rest of the class does when they feel themselves to be perfectly competent on their own – arithmetic exercises are an example. It is a feature of traditional education that when the teacher asks the class a question, she already has the 'correct' answer in mind. It is a type of 'guess what I'm thinking' teaching and gifted children sometimes give a purposefully 'wrong' answer to relieve the tedium. Informal child-centred teaching makes less demand on a child's capacity for patience, though perhaps that is something which gifted children are obliged to learn.

A problem often recognized by teachers is that a gifted child can be very lazy. The relatively effortless learning which keeps them ahead of their contemporaries in early childhood can bring about bad learning habits. Directed, concentrated learning of unwelcome subject matter shows up these bad habits. Sometimes gifted children have to learn how to learn in adolescence and breaking bad habits is far harder than acquiring good ones. It is important in the teaching of gifted children that they are not allowed to float through the syllabus without effort. It is not so much a matter of 'stretching', as of directed thought; independence of mind is fine in itself, but is not necessarily beneficial to an individual child in all aspects of education.

Because of their abilities, gifted young people are often faced with a multitude of educational options which they find difficulty in handling. They can do so many things so well. School counsellors are not a familiar sight in British schools, but they could be of great value to gifted pupils helping them to sort through the morasse of available subjects and possible choices of education. A school counsellor who has no subject axe to grind can act as negotiator when each teacher is claiming a gifted pupil for his own – a confusing situation for a child. Being generally gifted provides no guarantee of knowing what you want to do; the child with one special gift is very lucky in that respect. Educational guidance for the gifted is vitally important to their future and should be the concern of all the school staff who are involved with them.

## EDUCATION OF THE GIFTED

The familiar traditional methods at present used by schools to teach gifted children are in need of a radical rethink. In fact, as these children become more frequently recognized and treated as a special group, the means by which they are educated have increasingly been questioned. In general, though, they can benefit more from a change of approach than from a change of subject matter.

Most teaching procedures which are used at present act to control the rate of a pupil's progress through the syllabus and this control is usually related to age. Although a gifted child may be individually accelerated to a higher school class, the class as a whole will be treated as an age-group and so the gifted child often comes to be regarded as rather small for his 'age'. Acceleration and ability grouping are often used by schools as the most convenient administrative ways of dealing with gifted children. Which method is employed depends on the number of gifted children in the school; what is convenient for the school is not normally related to a particular child's previous progress, his abilities and his needs. In a truly child-centred (rather than administration-centred) school, all the children – as well as the gifted ones – would have these matters taken into consideration. But this is not an ideal world and practical difficulties often get in the way of how teachers would prefer to teach. It is possible, though, to administer a school so that the special abilities of gifted children may be at least recognized and allowed for and in such a way their educational development can be co-ordinated with the general curriculum and with the needs of the other children.

It might be thought that ordinary schools could not cope with very gifted children and indeed Hollingworth (1942) wrote 'In the ordinary elementary school situation children of IQ 140 waste half their time. Those above IQ 170 waste practically all their time'. Whatever the real situation may have been at that time, such a view received little or no support from the parents in my study. Of the 20 sample children of IQ 170, only one parent expressed anything less than complete satisfaction with their child's educational progress. As the means by which gifted children are taught are unlikely to be changed overnight, it is therefore heartening that such a high proportion of parents of gifted children in England are so satisfied with the school provision.

## Selective education

In Britain in 1946 the government of the time began a brave venture. It had been decided by the 1944 Education Act to direct children into forms of education which were suitable for their intellectual abilities and not governed by their parents' abilities to pay school fees. There was to be an examination which children took at about eleven years old, which became known as the eleven-plus. As a result of this, about 25% of children were sent to a grammar school where they had a good chance of going on to university or college; the remaining 75% or so went to a secondary modern school to be taught primarily more practical skills. There were also technical schools which were meant to supply the fields of industrial craft and design, but these never grew in number to any great extent. The system is presently being altered so that eventually all the neighbourhood children will go to their local 'comprehensive' school.

The initial shock of this system of selection was considerable. Some children who had expected to learn a trade and leave school at 15 years old like their parents were suddenly displaced at eleven into an academic education, in a school which had probably catered previously for their social superiors. An equally disconcerting effect on certain parents, who had not expected it, was when their child 'failed' the eleven-plus and was no longer permitted to attend the school which they had wanted. There was therefore a growth of small private schools following

255

this introduction of selection for those parents who could afford to make use of them.

Depending on the area in which the grammar school was situated and the number of places it had to offer, it was expected that a child would have to have a minimum IQ of about 120 to enter it. This selective system effectively creamed off the bright and gifted children into one form of education and the moderate and dull children into another. Although not considered so at the time, it was one of the biggest educational experiments ever devised in the world, before or since.

It had been the intention of the 1944 Act that the more intelligent but more impoverished and culture-bound child should be freed by the state and given a chance to succeed in the educated world. Thousands of bright youngsters did just that; the last four Prime Ministers of Britain have been grammar school pupils, for example. But the examination had too wide a margin of error for comfort and a very high proportion of children who were given this life chance still left school as soon as they could, with little to show for it. In fact, the selection effects were as much psycho-social as academic; pressure by parents on children rose steadily as the advantages of the free grammar school became more widely appreciated. Teachers began to drill children in intelligence tests at school, which resulted in anxiety symptoms such as sickness, nail biting and nightmares as the examination approached. Anxiety filled many homes and children were offered material gifts such as bicycles if they 'passed', though the majority of families took it in their stride. Many primary school teachers limited general teaching in order to train their pupils for particular kinds of tests or examinations which were used in selection. Thus, the curriculum was often narrowed down to the tests. Some children were heavily tutored so that they managed to pass the grammar school examination but were unhappy or unable to keep up later. Those who went to the secondary modern schools were often disappointed and resentful. They had been dubbed failures – at 11 years old – with the result that any further interest in educational progress was inhibited and they were often bored and rebellious.

In his review of research, in which he identified these unwelcome after-effects of eleven-plus selection, Vernon (1957) commented that:

'Such findings . . . probably reflect a more fundamental difference between families, which is closely bound up with social class mores. Nevertheless we must agree that selection for secondary schooling . . . tends to become a focussing point for such anxieties.'

In other words the socio-economic class system in education, which had been fairly static until this point, had received the intended jolt. But even in 1957, it was not entirely acceptable for Vernon to put it so bluntly. The effect on working class children in a hitherto middle class grammar school was often to promote a considerable reorientation to middle class attitudes, which caused some problems at home. There was very much less of a working class effect on middle class children, as rather fewer of them were sent to the grammar schools, and for those who failed the eleven-plus, there were always private schools. The upper classes, who are a statistically tiny proportion of the British population, went on as before sending their children to the schools which they had chosen themselves.

A. H. Halsey at Oxford, heading a research team on educational opportunity, has emerged with unexpected and as yet unpublished findings. He claims that the principal beneficiaries of state selective education were a so-called 'sunken middle class'. This was a group within the working class which included at least one close member of the family – usually the mother – who was objectively middle class in status or education. The attitudes and influence of the mother in promoting educational advancement, and indeed 'giftedness', in her children was also highlighted in my research; her influence is undoubtedly an extremely effective, if not the most significant, factor in a child's education. As is frequent in research, Halsey's team were concerned exclusively with the education of boys 'for economical reasons'; girls do not seem to feature in the education system. However, his research has shown that in spite of dramatic social change in Britain over the last 35 years, the social class structure has been shocked, but not seriously shaken.

There is considerable argument in Britain at the present time between those who think that gifted children should be removed from the public sector of education and sent to private schools at the taxpayers' expense, and those who see the gifted child's place as being within state education. The two assumptions underlying the first view are that we are able to identify these gifted children and that putting them into private schools will benefit them educationally. The arguments for private schools were summed up in a *Guardian* editorial:

'The thinking behind the proposition is indeed muddled – the most able it is alleged will be given intellectual opportunities denied them in the public sector, parental choice will be extended and an opportunity given for those drawn from different social classes to mix on equal terms' (The Guardian, July 25th, 1978).

The private schools and the parents concerned believe that gifted children would be given opportunities otherwise denied them and that there would be a healthy coming together of people from different social classes through a widening of parental choice – were the government to pay for the selected children. But where government grants have been awarded, the picture of who gets the free places is still not unlike that of the old eleven-plus selection. In 1972, figures (for Harrow Borough Council) covering the previous three years revealed that a third of all the places awarded came from the 10 primary schools situated in the more affluent areas of the borough; five schools in working class districts gained no places at all and a fifth of the places went to pupils already in the private sector. More precise evidence on the actual incomes of parents who received free places at private schools in the Harrow area showed that there was, in fact, very little social mixture. Most of the children who obtained them came from the more affluent areas, while the primary schools that served the working class areas of the borough and which contained the largest representation of ethnic minorities received no places at all.

The reason which parents most often give for choosing private education is the size of the classes in state schools and it is generally believed that private schools have smaller classes. Gifted children particularly could receive more of that special concern when there are less of them clamouring for the teacher's attention, while teachers also claim that children learn better in smaller classes.

However, results of research into the size of the 'normal' classroom are equivocal. Some studies have actually shown that children learn better in larger classes and it is very possible that class size is often made the scapegoat of the educational system. When children are not doing as well as adults think they should, then class size is blamed more readily than other less obvious educational conditions (Insel and Lindgren, 1978). My own research (p. 211) has shown that there was very little difference in average size of class between private and state schools involved in my sample, but there was much greater variation of class size in the private schools. Some of them did have smaller classes, but others had larger ones than in the state schools.

In a recent study into why parents preferred to send their sons to private schools, Bridgeman and Fox (1978) asked them what they thought they were buying. Middle class parents tended to choose the more 'meritocratic' of the private schools, believing that they gained an academic and intellectual advantage over the state schools. But upper class parents chose 'traditional schools', believing that they gained social advantage and what appeared to be a superior education by being associated with well known institutions. Most of the parents explained their choice in broad and not very well defined educational terms. Schools were seen as simply 'better', or as reflecting their own cultural values and identity to which they wished their sons to aspire. Whether these parents did actually buy what they believed their children to be receiving is a matter needing research, however.

## Problems and benefits of selective education

It is not possible to select some children to be treated differently from others without involving social values. But if it is to be done, with the best of intentions, then there is an urgent need for the people undertaking the selection to be fully aware of what they are doing and why. The tests used for this are usually reliable, though their validity is not always sure (as outlined in Chapter 3); psychologists are reworking and restandardizing them all the time and it is to be hoped that each new one, such as the British Intelligence Scales, will increase understanding of testing abilities. Children can be selected by parents, but as my research (Chapter 4) has shown, that is neither a reliable nor valid procedure, any more than is recommendation by teachers. Both parents and teachers are motivated in their choice of the gifted child by reasons which are personal to themselves – like identification and wishful thinking.

In the fine arts, gifted children are usually judged by a panel of experts, aesthetic performance not being considered amenable to objective testing. In a sense, being judged by a group of people as to whether you are better than the norm is not very different from the procedures used in a standardized test. It serves to retain the status quo and contains all the biases to which humans are prey. In other words, all forms of selection have their drawbacks and it is only through the constant search for better understanding of the ideas and procedures involved that the objectives may be achieved more fully as time goes on.

When children have been selected and then labelled as different from other children, they receive information about the sort of behaviour which is expected of them. If the message is to behave like a stereotype gifted child and the child acts accordingly, parents and school teachers will feel justified in their complaints. The circle has been set in motion.

Children who are academically more able and who go to special schools for such pupils will produce better examination results for these particular schools, but the education they receive is not necessarily the cause of the schools' good results; the motivation and expectations of the pupils have been found to be at least as effective. Some expensive private schools offer scholarships to gifted children. When they are accepted there, the parents believe their children are getting a better education and the school believes it is getting a child with award-winning potential which will reflect well on the school. All parties are satisfied then, but the losers are the schools from which the gifted children have been creamed off. Without their bright lively minds, a school is deprived of the top of the normal range of ability, does less well in examination results and is seen as a worse school.

The selection of gifted children for special education has led to the growth of specialisms, particularly in America. There are now schools for the gifted, special training for teachers of the gifted, advice centres on educational problems, etc. Although selection is less than sure and is often influenced by such matters as the socio-economic status of the child, gifted programmes are providing work and opportunities of acquiring expertise for staff in many parts of the USA. Most, if not all, of these schools are private and none yet exist in Britain, though one is proposed for Hampstead in North London. However, there are specialist music schools and several schools of dance and drama in this country.

One problem of specialist education is that it is sometimes lopsided. The attributes for which the child was selected in the first place are further encouraged so that her career possibilities become limited. Specialist schools are aware of this problem and try to see that the child does get a good all-round education, but children at these schools, of whatever sort, are separated from the rest of society for at least part of the day. There is the probability, as yet undocumented, that they have difficulty in adjusting to the non-specialist world. Being placed on a pedestal because of ability can lead to a devaluation of others' abilities and an overconcern with one's own. As such, selection may be said to be divisive of society.

Children may also be wrongly selected. As I discovered, not all children who are described as gifted by their parents were as intellectually able as they had been thought. Such children could be sent to schools for gifted children, since selection systems are less than perfect. Wrong selection brings about feelings of failure in a child, which may last for life if he is launched into a career for which he is not suited and from which, because of his educational bias, there is little opportunity to change. The only alternative may be to 'drop out' and leave the parent society.

However, the benefits of selective education for the gifted are considerable. Perhaps the best is the stimulating atmosphere which a child shares with his fellow pupils. It is usual in selective schools for pupils to be highly motivated and interested in what they are doing. Instead of in a normal school, where groups of pupils are pursuing different projects, a music school for example has all the pupils keen on music. The level of education in a selective school will be higher, either on a general intellectual level or in the specialist field of the school. Thus, the gifted child will indeed be 'stretched' in competition or co-operation with his ability peers and is unlikely to suffer from academic frustration.

The selection of their child confers vicarious merit on the parents, who are likely to respond positively with encouragement. The parents of children at selective schools are more likely to be involved in their child's education than those at a neighbourhood school. The school benefits from this general parental involvement, as does the child. As the cycle turns, the parents are more satisfied, the school benefits and the child benefits, at least in whatever he's been selected for. The losers are the neighbourhood school and, for the reasons outlined above, perhaps the child loses out on normal relationships with other people in the long run.

## Mixed ability teaching

It has been contended that gifted children in a normal heterogeneous classroom of children of mixed ability cannot discuss and debate with their intellectual peers. This intellectual exercise is therefore of little value to them, as the level at which they would have to function would be below their potential. Such a contention assumes that any child with ability above that of any other finds intellectual discourse between the two of them unfruitful. If a class genuinely reflects the whole range of abilities in children, it will contain those of a wide variety of abilities and experiences, which themselves are challenging in different ways.

The gifted child (or children) in such a class would have no need to feel isolated or superior, unless she has been made aware that this is expected of her. By the same subtle processes which adults use to make a child conform to racial prejudice or to realize that there are things which 'one does not do', a child can in his giftedness learn to be separate because he is 'better' than others. The more rigid the culture, the more different the deviant feels. Children of different racial origins can be seen huddling in separate groups in the school playground while the child who is neglected at home, whose clothes are torn and dirty, is as unacceptable as a child from another part of the country with a different accent. Giftedness as a label trails all sorts of unwarranted and unwelcome assumptions in its wake. Identifying the gifted child as different from his peers in order to give him a different education is in large part an ethical decision. But the immediate atmosphere of the school can mitigate this.

Ability grouping, though, even for part of the learning experience, can certainly make a difference to the education of gifted children and can help the teachers to help them. However, the mere grouping together of gifted pupils is not in itself enough; they need their own style and level of teaching if such separation is to be worthwhile. The benefit of ability grouping, bearing in mind its defects, is that it is possible for practically any school to do it, regardless of size or the age of pupils. But each school has to work out what is best in its own situation. In some schools where there is a particularly wide range of abilities amongst the children, there will be many possibilities for ability groupings, but perhaps in very small schools it would really be a waste of everyone's time; for instance, the one in my sample with only 20 pupils.

A recent government report in Britain (DES, 1978b) examined mixed ability comprehensive secondary schools all over the country. The inspectors made a two-year study of 22 schools in which most teaching is in mixed ability groups up to the end of the third year. This category is not actually representative of all comprehensive schools – only 9% of them in fact. They found that the teaching was traditional and pitched at a level which the teacher thought was appropriate to most of the class. Planning was inadequate and teachers' expectations were too low. Bright children lacked the stimulus of working with their peers so that examination work in the fourth or fifth years had to be unduly narrow and at high pressure to enable 'O' level candidates to make up lost ground.

However, when there were exceptionally good teachers, school timetables organized to produce small classes, generous supplies of teaching material and good ancillary help, mixed ability classes were seen as catering satisfactorily for all the children concerned. The less bright children undoubtedly gained from working with the bright ones and from seeing what they could achieve. They also gained by having access to materials and facilities sometimes denied to them in streamed schools; nowhere did they feel undervalued and there was observably high enthusiasm and motivation throughout.

Unfortunately, the report did not discuss issues such as the different results of long or short-term use of mixed ability teaching or how to achieve a satisfactory balance of advantage and disadvantage. Poor teaching, poor planning and assessment, or courses which bore the bright and baffle the stupid are no monopoly of schools with mixed ability teaching. The report states unequivocally that mixed ability teaching is harder; it requires more generous staffing and better training with better materials in order to be successful. But there was also a failure to point out how it might be done and how the drawbacks might be overcome. Nor does it describe how it managed to survey 'ability' over such a wide range of schools in two years or to judge success at all, and, since success was not actually defined, their evaluation of it under different schemes of teaching is questionable. The teachers in the survey had no training in mixed ability teaching and many of them said they did not really believe in it. Under such circumstances, the merits of this particular procedure could never be judged fairly and it is very sad that the one national survey of mixed ability teaching should falter in so many of its design aspects, making the results hazy and virtually unusable.

Another survey on mixed ability teaching carried out by the National Foundation for Educational Research in one comprehensive school found that gifted children did as well overall in mixed ability groups as they would have done in selected teaching groups (Newbold, 1977). The one subject in which brighter children did better when taught separately appeared to be English. The report found that teachers of academic subjects such as French and Mathematics were fearful that the standards achieved by the clever children would fall if they were taught in mixed ability classes. However, the study showed on the contrary that all the children did better, especially socially, and that it 'created a more healthy environment for the school as a whole'.

Teachers in this 2000 pupil co-educational school were particularly concerned about long-term effects on academic standards. Their doubts can only be answered by further follow-up studies over the years. This school has not been in existence in its present form for very long and it draws mostly on a middle class clientele; any research on just one school is bound to be limited by the individual characteristics of that institution. Mixed ability teaching did seem to work in this particular school, but that does not mean that it would work well for others.

# Acceleration

There are several methods by which the progress of a gifted child might be accelerated. She could simply be put up a class with children one or two years older than herself for all lessons. But the gifted child's learning ability does not lend itself to neat sequential ordering of tasks according to school class levels. Sometimes it may be necessary for her to stay with her own age-group for most of the lessons and be accelerated, say for Mathematics or French. Sometimes a gifted child may have to mark time for a while because it is simply not possible in a school of some hundreds of children to keep all of them intellectually stretched all of the time. There are some schools which will allow a gifted child to start education early. In Britain, where children begin 'proper' school in the year in which they are five, many children actually begin at four and a half so that early acceleration could mean starting school at three. The problem would not be quite so acute in America where normal admission to school begins at six years.

Acceleration within school has the problems of social adjustment, especially during adolescence. A sudden spurt into an older age-group can be a source of psychological stress to a gifted child. There are occasions when it is better to be intellectually less stretched and happier, than to fail at life and become an outcast from one's classmates. But acceleration is not a once-and-for-always act. A child could move for a certain length of time and then return to his class. A well organized school can be flexible and allow for a gifted child to be accelerated where and when it seems to be useful, while the rest of his school life carries on normally. But, above all, there must be continuity in education towards a specified goal.

# Independent study

The move towards independent study in primary school children has been in use now in Britain for many years under the heading of 'Project Work'. It certainly provides a means whereby the gifted child can pursue his own particular interest to any appropriate depth while at the same time remaining with his classmates. It enables a gifted child to explore to his heart's content within the ever-increasing amount and complexity of available knowledge.

Gifted children are capable of learning a great deal with relatively little teaching. They can benefit particularly from independent study, with assistance available when it is wanted. American schools, though, appear to make less use of this method than those in Britain, where it is an integral part of virtually every child's education in the state system. Whole or half school days are set aside for it and children are expected to continue their exploration out of school. Some schools allow pupils to attend to their independent studies throughout the day, in their spare time, while others set aside specific times for such work.

Independent study under supervision is truly individualization of education within an overall system; it need not even be related to the stated school syllabus. The prime necessity for a pupil is time, either in long or short spaces.

However, a well run, child-centred primary classroom has relatively few fixed lesson periods in a day. There are reading times, story times, playing times and project times which are all expected to be part of a child's partly self-organized education. A few secondary schools in Britain even operate on this system; the teachers who work in them like it and believe that it provides the best form of education for all pupils. But style of teaching is as yet very little researched as to its effectiveness. Critics of independent study say that, left to themselves, children do nothing useful.

Where a school works by team-teaching, individuals have much greater access to guidance in their individual projects. In this system about four to eight teachers work as a team, teaching together several 'classes' of children. The barriers between the school classes are broken down so that Miss Jones looks after those who want to read, Mr Phipps takes the model builders, Mrs Jackson supervises Arithmetic, etc., all at the same time. Children change subject and teacher almost at will – 'I've finished my reading; now I want to paint'. Again, critics say that this method encourages laziness but, as always, much of its success depends on the dedication and training of the teachers. It also depends very much on how soon the child is started in the way of choosing what to do next rather than being told. Children who come into the team-teaching situation late, say at eight years old, are confused by the relative freedom and seem to feel the need for more structure. Others, who have been accustomed to this freedom all their school lives, are resentful of the traditional pattern which they may encounter in a new school.

Obviously, pupils will vary in how they use the facilities available. It cannot be assumed that because a child is gifted, an open-plan, team-teaching situation will be fine. Gifted children, like others, require self-discipline and a willingness to accept guidance rather than didactic teaching. Teachers who are sensitive to pupils will be able to be more effective guides in helping them decide what to do. A gifted child may actually have the problem of too many exciting choices pressing for attention.

School facilities should be available for those who want them, even outside school hours. If only a few want to use them, special arrangements can be made, but when schools have been 'thrown open' to the community, it has been found that facilities are in great demand, at least during normal waking hours. When a child leaves school for college or university, it is expected that she will have developed skills of independent study. It is very strange, though, how divorced many secondary schools are from this practice so that many students spend much of their first year of higher education learning how to conduct independent study. If the value of a pupil's independent effort is seen to be as great as the value of the work set by the teacher, then time will be found for it. In the case of gifted children, it must certainly be found as they need the growing space.

## Enrichment

The fruitfulness of any type of education is largely dependent on how it is received. What may appear as high quality or enriched education to one group, say the local education authority, may be merely filling in time for another group - the school leavers. Where education is inappropriate or unwelcome, it is clearly wasteful of resources. Enrichment of the curriculum is usually taken to mean the inclusion of subject matter which does not fall into the category of basic education, such as music or world affairs. But this enrichment in a normal school rarely occupies a significant status in relation to more mundane learning. Too often, for example, class singing and water colouring or painting at the desk are the sum total of aesthetic activities. Enrichment is particularly important for the potentially talented in such subjects, but it is also a cause for concern in relation to all children. The sooner the open mind and supple fingers of a young child begin to practise the skills of an art, the finer her technique will become over time.

An enriched curriculum for the gifted child does not mean that the basic subject teaching should aim at a higher level; it must rather provide a deeper, broader and more diversified education. Resources have to be both material and human in order that the child of high ability can pursue his interests to the full extent. However, the use of extra resources should not be restricted to the high achiever. They should be available for the unidentified gifted child to discover and so designed that the less able child can make use of them at perhaps a more superficial level.

The enrichment of normal school education does not need to take place in school buildings or in school houses. Teachers' centres, for example, are open in the evenings and often contain a wealth of extra-curricular material for teachers to study. Gifted children can benefit from using teachers' centres and teachers can benefit from the children's presence. For children who can benefit from an extended school day and teachers who would like to extend their knowledge of gifted children, the combination would work well.

Various schools and local education authorities have experimented with ideas of enrichment. A school may call it a 'hobbies' afternoon or schedule individual work into its time-table. Some bring in part-time 'enriching' staff, i.e. specialists who are probably additional to normal staffing ratios. Music and dance, for example, have long been taught in schools by peripatetic teachers. It is not too difficult for an educational administration to extend the idea to basic subjects such as Biology or English. The problem is either one of money or of willingness to recognize the educational situation of the gifted child. Staff can be interchanged between primary and secondary schools, which would enable their different skills to be shared and would be attractive to the teachers. More use can also be made of parents with special skills than is at present normal in British schools. It would even be possible to set up at very little cost a regional co-ordination scheme of willing parents.

Enrichment can be part-time, as in the Brentwood Experiment (Bridges, 1969) in which gifted children were bussed around for their enrichment like a football team going for practice. Bridges stated that few educationists have felt the need for such an activity because there is a basic, unexamined assumption that each school is self-sufficient, that it can cater for all the educational needs of all its pupils. He suggests that gifted children be collected up and transported, preferably for a day or a week at a time, to another school or centre where the extra programme can be given. In practice, the experiment went extremely well with the co-operation of parents and students as guardians of the children in their journeyings.

The unfortunate aspect of enrichment in one school is that one cannot continue to add to the curriculum indefinitely without taking something away. Days are limited in length and even gifted children are limited in energy and enthusiasm. The pick-and-choose, 'supermarket' approach to the curriculum can be confusing and overwhelming. Children need choice, but the more choice there is, the more supervision they need in making sure that the essentials of education are attended to. There is also the possibility that children will be tempted to flit from choice to choice so that a steady building up of standards is difficult to organize.

As with all education, a policy of enrichment for gifted children must be clear and explicit as to what is being enriched and to what purpose. Individual approaches by children to the subjects under consideration must be taken into account when preparing the teaching material. Enrichment should not be an extension of school work, but exercises and experiments in thinking and feeling which are separate from the basic school curriculum. Progress in enrichment has to be evaluated too in order to be seen to be related to what has been done and to decide what to do next. The possibilities of extended education for the gifted, inherent in the concept of enrichment, are limitless and can take place in normal schools with normal teachers.

## Teachers

The reasons why people become teachers are as varied as, for example, security, long holidays, it's all they 'know', and a real desire to teach. In general, prospective teachers have themselves enjoyed being taught and are very often the children of teachers. As they are unlikely to have had much experience of the outside world, the profession is sometimes said to be overly concerned with academic matters and inward looking which, in turn, has a narrowing effect on what is taught in schools.

The question most often raised about teachers of the gifted is – do they have to be gifted themselves? In IQ terms, most teachers probably are gifted; that is they will be found in the top 2% of the population. But they will not have had special education for teaching the top 0.05% of children or necessarily be aware of and sympathetic to them. Many teachers suffer from a degree of artistic, practical, physical, creative and sensitivity atrophy, brought about by their own training of continual paper and pencil examinations. Although this is interspersed with bouts of teaching practice, it is the examinations which are nearly always the most important for their final qualifications. Before teachers can enjoy teaching children, they have to rediscover their own latent learning pleasure and rusty abilities.

Educational psychology is an integral part of all teacher training programmes, but it is rarely learnt in a useful form, being overburdened with theory and academically acceptable topics which are not always appropriate to teachers' needs. Even with a basic understanding of child development, teachers very often emerge from their training with little scientific basis for judging the children in their care unless their own course has made a speciality of assessment procedures. It is possible for teachers to become qualified without the simplest understanding of statistics, such as the possible meanings of a comparison of childrens' scores on an achievement test. Understanding and coping with exceptional children, including gifted children, is most frequently considered to be the preserve of specialists, while more serious children's problems must wait for the educational psychologist. But in fact, teachers are in the most favourable position to notice a child who is gifted or who is in emotional difficulty; in most circumstances, they should be able to help without recourse to a specialist.

A teacher's self-understanding of her own strengths and weaknesses is the first step towards understanding others. Students who, as part of their training, are able to make use of experiential group training sessions or practice their personal interactions with a video-tape camera as feed-back, will be more aware both of themselves and others. They will also be better prepared for the position of developmental guide with children, rather than that of old-style didactic teacher. Teachers are particularly responsible for the emotional and social development of their very young pupils and exceptional children are particularly in need of this non-family guidance. It would be as well if teachers were universally trained for this counselling/teaching aspect of their work.

Teachers come from a predominantly aspiring middle class background as a result of processes in which they have been sorted through the educational system, as well as the traditional attitudes towards teaching, as a route to the white collar' life. In colleges of education, the women tend to come from a higher social class than men. Not surprisingly, teachers generally value the educational system which has benefited them and this attitude affects both their own aspirations and their perception of the ways in which individual pupils fit into the system they know. Most teachers speak to their pupils in a form of English which is considered to be grammatically correct and suitable for imitation. Pupils whose morals, manners and out-of-school activities are patently not in the approved style are likely to be at odds with the teacher's ideas of the 'best' ways of living. Research results show that teachers are more easily able to identify with and encourage pupils from higher social classes than themselves.

In American schools which have been desegregated, these teachers' attitudes are particularly harmful to gifted minority children. Even in a desegregated school they are likely to remain a minority, the schools from which they have come are likely to be seen as inferior and their potential for future performance seen as limited at a fairly low level. All too often, the result has been a resegregation through grouping and tracking procedures so that the poor, the black and the non-English-speaking are relegated into the slower, non-academic programmes which are basically inferior in quality. The gifted and talented among these 'homogeneous' minority groups are particularly vulnerable. The same thing happens in Britain to immigrant children who find themselves in remedial education because of their poor English, although their ability is very varied.

Peer values, social position and achievement motivation limit the extent to which a child may manifest his giftedness in a situation where his teacher perceives his potential as low. The possibility of this false situation existing is accepted by certain schools, who attempt to avoid it by careful organization. But the best intentions can be subverted in the classrooms by teachers who are unable to relate either themselves personally or their teaching procedures to the needs of gifted children from unpromising backgrounds.

To teach gifted children, a teacher must have a thorough mastery of her subject area and be a particularly bright and stimulating guide. It is very difficult to keep just one step ahead of gifted children; the truth is always preferable. To say 'I don't know; let's find out' is not acceptable for teachers in all cultures, but it is essential in a teacher's relationship with gifted pupils. Where the teacher feels the need to be seen to be 'all knowing' and invincible, then she should question her decision to work with gifted children. Is she seeking some kind of proof of her own abilities? Knowing your own limitations is a large part of knowing yourself. Briefly, teachers of gifted children should be aware of themselves and others, bright (but not necessarily gifted), knowledgeable and keen. The combination of a gifted child and such a gifted teacher must be extremely satisfactory and productive to all concerned.

## Teaching gifted children

It is not the concern of this book to detail specific ways by which gifted children may exercise their special gifts. The techniques and material that may be used in the education of these children are still in the process of development and testing and the results of this work are now emerging more frequently into print. The emphasis of this book, however, has been on pointing out potentially useful routes in the education of gifted children, as indicated by my own research and that of others.

All good teaching involves showing pupils how to learn, but in order to do this, a teacher must first be aware of and be able to communicate the nature and processes of learning. Gifted children, like other children, can acquire faulty learning techniques which will persist with them through life.

Teaching gifted children is obviously more than just stimulating and stretching an already active, seeking mind. To get the most out of learning, the gifted child is particularly well placed to know what she is aiming for and to appreciate how well she is doing. Young children need short-term goals but, as they get older, goals or end-products of learning become more diffuse and their values can be recognized in a wider context than that of immediate reward. Gifted children are less happy than most with snippets of syllabus being handed out to them. The pattern of learning which they are to pursue is more acceptable as a whole, so that each child can tackle particular aspects of it in their own personal way - not always that most appealing to the teacher. Educational objectives such as those of Bloom are designed to be used by teachers, but need not be confined to them. Exercises in the setting up of objectives in learning are in fact of great value both to gifted pupils and to teachers.

Effective learning, especially for young gifted children, must be meaningful in terms of experiences which are acceptable to the child according to his competence, interests and background. Teaching involves structuring of learning in such a way that the child can absorb it but also be creative in the learning process. Although creativity might be thought of as an end-product of learning, it is also that continuing part of the process which enables learning to be flexible so that it may be used in a wide variety of ways. Discovery methods of learning make hard work for the teacher; she is then not a watcher on someone else's shore, but an active participant in the discovery and creation of new understanding. Perhaps it is the ability to be at once a teacher and a pupil, to be as excited as a child at the rediscovery of simple learning, that requires a high degree of empathy and a true love of teaching.

It has always been the situation in the classroom that the teacher has been responsible for the product of learning rather than the process. This emphasis on the end-product calls for the presentation of the subject matter in some form of logical progression, normally from simple to complex, from singular to plural and whenever possible in chronological order. But gifted children may not find this form of teaching best suited to their abilities. They may have the facility to 'skip' parts of the logical process while a teacher may be continuing to explain a progression in the time-honoured manner which is actually irrelevant to the thinking processes of a gifted child. It is at this point that the gifted child may experience boredom or impatience; she is not then being held back by the others in the class, but by the inappropriate style of teaching.

Barbe and Frierson (1975) describe two styles of teaching – product-orientated, which they consider suitable for normal pupils, and process-orientated, which they believe is appropriate for gifted pupils. My contention, however, is that not only is process-orientated teaching better for gifted children, but for all children. When learning to learn is given a higher value than the learning of information, then the educational system will have made a big step in the direction of enabling children to be autonomous students (in the general sense) for life. By encouraging the exploratory aspects of learning, its excitement and inherent satisfaction can be generalized into an approach to all life experiences; learning then is not associated only with school and the classroom, but becomes a part of living.

The concept of teaching which is concerned with learning to learn necessitates changes in teaching style from traditional to explanatory. The teacher must be skilled at her profession in order to continue maintaining enthusiasm for knowledge. Lessons have to be planned in these terms and not in the traditional terms of logical sequence, while the teacher remains aware and able to take action when old habits of thought inhibit the new learning. Above all, teachers must be 'with' the pupil; empathy is not a once-and-for-all facility; it can be helped along and deepened for any teacher. The teacher must also be ready to learn and indeed act as a model herself, though exploratory teaching should never be used as a means of promotion. Evaluation is part of the learning to learn procedure; without regular checking, the pupil cannot be sure where he is or where he is going. It is, however, a matter for pupil and teacher to sort out together.

As with all teaching, the exploratory style has its limitations but these are not of the teacher's mind. They may be due to limitations for pupils of resources such as libraries or home conditions. Pupils themselves are limited in their life experiences, both by their circumstances and their ages. Gifted children can jump to conclusions by a process of brilliant mental leaps, which are wrong because of lack of information. In a reassuring 'safe' exploratory classroom, mistakes are part of the process of learning; they are not 'failures'. The teacher of the gifted child is in a particularly important position – not there to demonstrate her superior knowledge or to show what a good actress she is, but to enable children to grope and leap towards understanding. It is important that the bounds of that understanding are determined by the characteristics of the pupils, not of the teacher or the school.

## Self-help groups

Over the last 20 years or so there has been a rapid increase in the number and variety of self-help and interest groups, which now form a significant feature of contemporary society. It does not need sociologists, psychologists, historians or priests to point out that mutual assistance in common problems has always been a feature of human life. But present day groups of this kind have recognized characteristics and ways of functioning, which are now becoming very well documented and classified. The National Association for Gifted Children (UK) is such a group.

Self-help groups most typically see themselves as fellowships, while putting great stress on the common problem, position or circumstances which bring the members together, i.e. being in the same boat. This means first of all understanding the problems of others, or knowing what it is like in this case to be the parent of a gifted child. It is said that only those experiencing the problem can really understand, and this understanding, based on common experiences, produces the necessary common bond of mutual interest and the common desire to do something about a particular problem. But in order to be a member of the group, it is essential to recognize that the difficulty exists. Many groups say that the relief experienced on first sharing the problem is their members' single most important experience. To be a member of the National Association for Gifted Children (NAGC) is to recognize that giftedness can be a problem and to have expressed a desire to help with it.

Once the group is formed and the common difficulties have been described, the first move is to share information and attempt practical assistance. This may be by money or equipment or, as with the NAGC, by advice, counselling and activities. It may also be by providing a social identity so that parents, say of gifted children, may accept their 'usuality' within their own group. Friendships and relationships within a self-help group are immensely important to its functioning; they can be encouraged formally, but seem to develop better through informal social activities. Friendship fosters a feeling that help and understanding are always available as distinct from the kind of institutionalized help, such as that of a medical doctor, which has to be applied for. Nor is there specialized knowledge which is retained by the helper and denied to the helped in this situation, though professional helpers such as psychologists do give their services to the NAGC.

Although self-help groups exist most obviously for the benefit of their members, most are also committed to changing the attitudes and behaviours of non-members towards the objects of their concern. In this way, such groups try to affect the population as a whole. A group may appear to be independent, if not even anti-society, but it is in fact an integral part of the society in which it operates. This aspect of working from within society has important implications for the group in respect of its attitude to deviance and to the relevant existing systems which the group wants to change. It is because groups usually function in a similar manner to the larger society from which they come that their systems of operation are found to be very similar. Hence, a traditional hierarchy of authority can emerge with accompanying cliques, as well as reward and punishment for members in relation to membership of the group. Self-help groups are actually effective in controlling their members by a judicious mixture of commitment and sanction.

Some groups are inward-looking, seeking entirely to help their members, while others are more concerned with changing the external order of things. A group may begin as an organization to help its members but broaden its scope, becoming involved in legislation and in promoting the understanding of social issues. In a major survey, Steinman and Traunstein (1976) found that almost three-quarters of the self-help organizations they studied wanted to change both the public and their own membership's image of their condition from being 'deviant' to being 'different'. However, despite their efforts to the contrary, campaigning groups may serve only to reinforce the stereotype that they are out to change. In order to campaign, the group needs publicity, which can be a double-edged sword; it seems almost inevitable that the group's case will be overstated, sometimes to the point of ludicrousness. Distorted presentation by the media can also affect the seriousness and credibility of the cause, perhaps serving to put off potential members or to affect the self-image of those who have already joined.

Organizations which exist to promote the wellbeing of gifted children are not exempt from the dynamics of the self-help group. The organization may be attempting to show the gifted as different not deviant, but in order to state their cause for concern, they must show how giftedness is likely to result in distress. It is an essential part of the argument for the recognition of gifted children as a case for special treatment that to be gifted in a mediocre world is to be in a stressful situation.

## SYNTHESIS

The research project which I have outlined in this book was intended to examine the life situations of gifted children. Though they function on a different intellectual and educational level from normal children of the same age, they are part of our community and it is the responsibility of everyone to see that they are accepted as such and that their needs are adequately supplied from our common resources.

Much of the concern which is now being shown for the recognition and education of the gifted child, both in Britain and America, is due to voluntary associations of parents. However, this brings with it the problem that voluntary organizations attract particular kinds of parents and children. The adults who run the activities of these societies tend to become so deeply involved in providing for the specialized needs of gifted children that they generalize too completely from those that they know well. Parents have a lot to teach teachers and psychologists from their own experiences, but they lack the undoubted advantages of professional expertise and freedom from deep personal involvement. Indeed, were parents to be as detached from their children as scientists, the parent–child relationship would necessarily suffer.

Certain basic themes have appeared throughout the book. Firstly, there is the inadequacy of previous research on gifted children; the Gulbenkian project is probably the first to survey gifted children in their home and school environments. Another theme is the beneficial effect of the recognition of gifted children as children, rather than stereotypes, but this recognition still has to be made general. Much research and published information about gifted children has concentrated on the minority who are disturbed and this in itself has served to accentuate their problems. My research, however, was designed to take a wider view, including gifted children who had not been labelled with the behavioural attributes of the stereotype.

Another main theme has been the vital importance of the early years in a child's life, particularly in relation to the development of behaviour, achievement and relationships with other people. If gifted children could be identified at an early age, those who needed it could be given extra help. The level of provision for gifted children seems to depend mainly on where a child happens to live and communication between parents and teachers also seems to be largely fortuitous. Sometimes teachers resent the parental belief that their child is gifted, but on the other hand some parents find it difficult to accept the teacher's professional judgement that any particular form of education is suitable for their child.

There are gifted children who are finding life difficult and for whom a full psychological assessment would be a great help. But the majority of parents and teachers need more general information about gifted children. They need to know what is being provided by the local education authority and why, but some schools refuse to discuss the matter with parents at all.

Attitudes towards gifted children are a reflection of their acceptance as a group within society. Special recognition or help for the gifted in any form are unlikely to thrive in times of financial stringency, though quite a number of programmes seem to be going ahead at the moment, both in Britain and America. The insights gained from working with these special children and the new techniques based on increased knowledge of them will have much wider application, since these children do not differ in kind from others but show in varying degrees all the difficulties and problems faced by the normal child. It is particularly important that regular teachers should be made aware of the presence of gifted children in their classrooms and that others with suitable training should be available for enrichment or other special teaching.

## The educational needs of gifted children

As psychologists and educators have begun to realize the great complexity of ability in children as a whole, education has become more child-centred, less teacher-centred, and more humane. The complexities of gifted children's abilities are even more difficult to provide for than those of normal children. But it is difficult to know whether there is a real difference between the merely bright and the gifted and how or whether to adjust their education accordingly. Recently in Britain the Warnock Report (DES, 1978a) has recommended that local education authorities should operate procedures for monitoring whole age-groups of children at least three or four times during their school life, in order to identify children with special educational needs, though such monitoring would not necessarily involve testing. Certainly, teachers should be trained to look for and recognize gifted children since early opportunities are particularly important for the development of talent.

But it is also important to remember that a gifted child is indeed a child and not some other being in the guise of a child. Children want to be like other children and to isolate the gifted because of their potential learning power is to do them a disservice. The quality of their lives, as well as the life of the society they live in depends on the contributions of the entire community, not just on those of an elite.

As the age of technology moves swiftly into its microprocessing phase so that fewer than ever low-skilled workers are needed, future ways of improving the life of the Developed World must lie in the area of social development. When everything that can be automated is controlled by relatively few people, the gifted amongst us – those who are able to think and communicate at a high level – will be even more important than at present. It is consequently of vital importance to all our futures that the gifted be well adjusted and in tune with their fellow humans. During the expansion of automation it is gifted adults who guide its growth and our present gifted children who will take over this guidance. As satisfaction in life becomes less centred on work, it can only come from human relationships, as it has begun to do already. The gifted, with their heightened perception and ability, will then become most valuable to society if these assets can be made available for the benefit of people generally.

It is especially in aesthetic activities that the gifted need to be able to communicate fluently. Although there are many educationalists who disapprove of segregating gifted children in general, they usually concede that the aesthetically gifted should go to specialist schools. A unique study which questioned outstanding performers in music and ballet found that the artistes were specific in recommending separate education for ballet dancers but not for musicians – either singers or instrument players (Povey, 1975). One of the sample musicians even said that 'to educate them separately often leads to a lack of "human" sympathies which can reflect in their music'. Such a statement, although from a successful musician's point of view, seems to sum up the dangers of poor communication engendered in the separating of gifted children in general from their fellows.

Over-emphasis on academic, intellectual learning tends to have a side-effect, even for the gifted, of leading to superficial verbalization which is without real personal meaning; in the same manner, a toddler's 'clever' remarks are delighted in by parents but are usually imitative and not derived from the child's own experiences. A gifted child is as happy to obtain approval as any other, though of course she is better at presenting evidence for it, for instance by obtaining good marks in school.

A preoccupation with excellence, though, can turn sour because it is meaningless to the child, except in terms of adult approval. This can result in negative attitudes towards school, which appear either as apathy or misbehaviour. Such distressing behaviour in gifted children can often be related to a failure of the educational system responsible for them and unsuitability of the educational goals set for them. In the long years of education in which they are involved, educational satisfaction has to be ensured for them from active participation and from solving meaningful and challenging problems. It is not the product or mark which is really important in the long run but the means by which this has been obtained. To help them in this process, gifted children need well adjusted teachers, who are open to new experiences and new learning themselves and who can give them encouragement, challenge and guidance at least as much as to other children.

Education in schools is still tied at present to a form of society which is past. This is inevitable to some extent, as a changing society moves ahead of those responsible for the curriculum. But even so, many of the bases on which Western education was founded are no longer there. The old traditions of reason and logic, within the context of old knowledge, are slowly being undermined by 'deviant' ideas and by the acceptance of children as emotional beings. There has never before been a time of more considered thinking about education, even though its practice has so far changed relatively little. Schoolchildren's learning is still governed ultimately by university entrance requirements and work opportunities, not by what is in the best interests of the individual children.

The fixed concepts and compartmentalized ways of thinking into which most children are induced in school are not actually beneficial to them or to the rest of society now. Postman and Weingartner (1975) sum up the new intellectual strategies for the nuclear and space age which are applicable in all dimensions of human activity. They include such concepts as 'relativity, probability contingency, uncertainty, function, structure as process, multiple causality (or non-causality), nonsymmetrical relationships, degrees of difference and incongruity (or simultaneously appropriate difference)'. These concepts and others which are implicit and contingent upon them are the ingredients for change, in ways that complement the new environmental demands. It is gifted children who are best equipped to learn the appropriate ways of thinking in order to deal more effectively with the future. These children must be mentally flexible and well adjusted, able to face uncertainty without distress and to formulate new meanings and processes from the evidence available. If gifted children are not up to this challenge because of their implied greater delicacy of mind, then no-one will be. The process of adaptation to new circumstances in humans require courage, stability and skill. This is what I believe gifted children have in abundance. But if all we can offer them is the superficial pursuit of traditional values, they will not be suitably equipped for the task. The provision of a personally meaningful and contemporary education for our gifted children is vitally important for all of us.

# Bibliography

Abroms, K.I., Moely, B.E., Gollin, J.B., and Kennedy, M. (1979). A developmental study of intellectually gifted pre-school children and their relationships to measures of psychosocial giftedness. Presented at the *Third World Conference for Gifted and Talented Chilren*, July, Jerusalem.

Anastasi, A. (1958). *Differential Psychology*. (New York: Macmillan).

Bandura, A. (1967). The role of modelling processes in personality development. In *The Young Child: Reviews of Research*. (National Association for the Education of Young Children). Reprinted in T.M. Roley, R.A. Lockhart, and D.M. Merrick (eds). *Contemporary Readings in Psychology*. (New York: Harper and Row).

Bandura, A. (1969). Social learning theory of identification processes. In David A. Goslin (ed.). *Handbook of Socialisation Theory and Research*. (Chicago: Rand McNally).

Bandura, A., and Walters, R.H. (1963). *Social Learning and Personality Development*. (New York: Holt, Rinehart and Winston).

Bandura, A., Grusec, J.E. and Menlove, F.L. (1967). Vicarious extinction of avoidance behaviour. *Journal of Personality and Social Psychology*, **5**, 16–23.

Barbe, W.B. and Frierson, E.C. (1975). Teaching the gifted – a new frame of reference. In W.B. Barbe and J.S. Renzulli (eds.). *Psychology and Education of the Gifted*. (New York: John Wiley).

Barry, H. III, Bacon, M.K., and Child, I.L. (1957). A cross-cultural survey of some sex differences in socialisation. *Journal of Abnormal and Social Psychology*, **55**, 327–332.

Bayley, N. (1957). Data on the growth of intelligence between 16 and 21 years as meaured by the Wechsler-Bellevue Scale. *Journal of Genetic Psychology*, **90**, 3–15.

Beez, W.V. (1968). Influence of biassed psychological reports on teacher behaviour and performance. Proceedings of *76th Annual Convention of the American Psychological Society No. 3*.

Bell, S.M. and Ainsworth, M.D.S. (1972). Infant crying and maternal responsiveness. *Child Development*, **43**, 4, 1170–1180

Belmont, L. and Marolla, F.A. (1973). Birth order, family size and intelligence. *Science*, **182**, 1096–1101.

Bennett, S.N. (1976). *Teaching Styles and Pupil Progress*. (London: Open Books).

Berg, I. (1970). *Education and Jobs: The Great Training Robbery*. (London: Penguin).

Bernstein, B. (1960). Language and social class. *British Journal of Social Psychology*, **2**, 311–326

Bernstein, B. (1972). *Class, Codes and Control*. (London: Routledge and Kegan Paul).

Bettelheim, B. (1969). *The Children of the Dream*. (New York: Macmillan).

## Bibliography

Bonsall, M. and Stefflre, U.J. (1955). The temperament of gifted children. *California Journal of Educational Research*, **6**, 162–165.

Boocock, S. (1972). *An Introduction to the Sociology of Learning*. (Boston: Houghton Mifflin).

Bowlby, J. (1951). *Maternal Care and Mental Health*. (Geneva: World Health Organisation).

Brazelton, T.B. (1975). Mother infant reciprocity. In M.H. Klaus, T. Leger and M.A. Trause (eds.). *Maternal Attachment and Mothering Disorders: A Round Table*. (New Brunswick: Johnson and Johnson).

Bridgeman, T. and Fox, I. (1978). Why people choose private schools. *New Society*, **44**, 702–705.

Bridges, S. (ed.). (1969). *Gifted Children and the Brentwood Experiment*. (London: Pitman).

Bridges, S. (1973). *IQ-150*. (London: Priory Press).

Bronfenbrenner, U. (1974). The origins of alienation. *Scientific American*, **231**, 53–61.

Brown, G.W. and Harris, T. (1978). *The Social Origins of Depression*. (London: Tavistock).

Burt, C. (1963). Is intelligence distributed normally? *British Journal of Statistical Psychology*, **16**, 175–190.

Cattell, R.B. and Cattell, M.D. (1973). *High School Personality Questionnaire*. (Illinois: Institute for Personality and Ability Testing).

Cazden, C.B. (1970). The neglected situation in child language research and education. In F. Williams (ed.). *Language and Poverty*, pp. 81–101. (Chicago: Markham Publishing Co.)

Chaikin, A.E., Sigler and Derlega, U. (1974). Non-verbal mediators of teacher expectancy effects. *Journal of Personality and Social Psychology*, **30**, 144–149.

Child, Dennis. (1977). Affective influences on academic performance. Inaugural lecture, University of Newcastle-upon-Tyne.

Child, I. (1954). Socialisation. In G. Lindsay (ed.). *Handbook of Social Psychology*. (Reading, Mass: Addison-Wesley).

Claiborn, W.L. (1969). Expectancy effects in the classroom; a failure to replicate. *Journal of Educational Psychology*, **60**, 377–383.

Clark, M.M. (1976). *Young Fluent Readers*. (London: Heinemann Educational Books).

Clarke, Ann and Clarke, A.D.B. (1976). *Early Experience: Myth and Evidence*. (London: Open Books).

Coan, R.W. and Cattell, R.B. (1976). *Early-School Personality Questionnaire*. (Champaign, Ill: IPAT).

Coleman, J.S. (1961). *The Adolescent Society*. (New York: Free Press).

Cowen, E.L., Penderson, A., Babigan, H., Izzo, L.D. and Trost, M.A. (1973). Long-term follow-up of early detected vulnerable children. *Journal of Consulting and Clinical Psychology*, **41**, 438–446.

Cox, Catherine Morris. (1926). The early mental traits of three hundred geniuses. In Louis Terman (ed.). *Genetic Studies of Genius*. (California: Stanford University Press).

Cronbach, L.J. (1964). *Essentials of Psychological Testing*. (London: Harper and Row).

Cronin, J., Daniels, N., Hurley, A., Kroch, A. and Webber, R. (1975). Race, class and intelligence: a critical look at the IQ controversy. *International Journal of Mental Health*, **3**, 46–132.

Cullen, K. (1969). *School and Family*. (Dublin: Cahill).

Davie, R., Butler, N. and Goldstein, H. (1972). *From birth to seven. A report of the National Child Development Study*. (London: Longmans).

Department of Education and Science (1967). *Children and Their Primary Schools*. (Plowden Report). (London: HMSO).

Department of Education and Science (1977). *Gifted Children in Middle and Comprehensive Schools*. (London: HMSO).

Department of Education and Science (1978a). *Special Educational Needs.* Report of the Committee of Enquiry into the Education of Handicapped Children and Young People. (Warnock Report) (London: HMSO).

Department of Education and Science (1978b). *Mixed Ability Work in Comprehensive Schools.* (London: HMSO).

Douglas, J.B.W. (1964). *Home and School.* (London: Panther).

Douglas, J.B.W. (1968). *All Our Future.* (London: Peter Davies).

Douglas, J.B.W. (1975). Early hospital admissions and later disturbances of behaviour and learning. *Developmental Medicine and Child Neurology,* 17, 456-80.

Drummond *et al.* (1976). Stability of self-concepts of elementary school children in two types of classroom organisation. *Elementary School Guidance and Counselling,* 10, 4 May.

Dunstan, J. (1977). *Paths to Excellence and the Soviet School.* (Windsor: NFER).

Durkheim, E. (1952). *Suicide: A Study in Sociology.* (London: Routledge).

Durkin, D. (1966). *Children Who Read Early.* (New York: Teachers' College Press).

Dwyer, C.A. (1963). Sex differences in reading. *Review of Educational Research,* 43, 455.

Edwards, A.L. (1969). *Experimental Design in Psychological Research.* (New York: Holt, Rinehart and Winston).

Elliott, C. (1974). Intelligence and the British Intelligence Scale. *Bulletin of the British Psychological Society,* 27, 313-17.

Eysenck, H.J. (1973). *The Inequality of Man.* (London: Temple Smith).

Ferri, E. (1976). *Growing Up in a One-Parent Family.* (Windsor: NFER).

Finn, J.D. (1972). Expectations and the educational environment. *Review of Educational Research,* 42, 3.

Ford, J. (1969). *Social Class and the Comprehensive School.* (London: Routledge and Kegan Paul).

Freeman, Joan. (1973). Attitudes of secondary school teachers towards prospective school counsellors. *British Journal of Guidance and Counselling,* 1, 79-84.

Freeman, Joan. (1974). Musical and artistic talent in children. *Psychology of Music,* 2, 5-12.

Freeman, Joan. (1975). *In and Out of School.* (London: Methuen).

Freeman, Joan. (1976a). The Gulbenkian Project on gifted children. In J. Gibson and P. Chennels (eds.). *Gifted Children - Looking to their Future.* (London: Latimer).

Freeman, Joan (1976b). Developmental influences on children's perception. *Educational Research,* 19 (1), 69-75.

Freeman, Joan. (1977). Social factors in aesthetic talent. *Research in Education,* 17, 63-76.

Freeman, J., Butcher, H.J. and Christie, T. (1968). *Creativity: a Selective View of Research.* (London: Society for Research into Higher Education).

Freud, E., Freud, L. and Grubrick-Simitis, I. (eds.) (1978). *Sigmund Freud. His Life in Pictures and Words.* (London: Andre Deutsch).

Fromm, E. (1941). *Escape from Freedom.* (London: Holt, Rinehart and Winston).

Furneaux, Barbara. (1976). *The Special Child.* (England: Penguin Education Specials).

Gallagher, J.J. (1975). Characteristics of gifted children: a research summary. In W.B. Barbe and S. Renzulli (eds.). *Psychology and Education of the Gifted.* (New York: John Wiley).

Galton, F. (1869). *Hereditary Genius.* (London: Macmillan).

Garai, J.E. and Scheinfeld, A. (1968). Sex differences in mental and behaviour traits. *Genetic Psychology Monographs,* 77, 169-299.

Gauld, Alan and Shotter, John. (1977). *Human Action and its Psychological Investigation.* (London: Routledge and Kegan Paul).

Gesell, A. (1950). *The First Five Years of Life.* (London: Methuen).

Gesell, A., Ilg, F.L. and Ames, L.B. (1965). *The Child From Five to Ten.* (London: Hamish Hamilton).

# Bibliography

Getzels, J.W. and Jackson, P.W. (1962). *Creativity and Intelligence: Explorations with Gifted Children.* (New York: John Wiley).

Gibson, J. and Chennells, P. (eds.) (1976). *Gifted Children: Looking to their Future.* (London: Latimer).

Goldstein, H. (1971). Factors influencing the height of 7-year-old children: Results from the National Child Development Study. *Human Biology,* **43**, 553-568.

Goodenough, Florence. (1926). *Measurement of Intelligence by Drawings.* (New York: World Book Co.).

Goslin, D.A. (1963). *The Search for Ability.* (New York: Russell Sage Foundation).

Graham, P.J. (1975). Environmental influences on psychosocial development. *International Journal of Mental Health,* **6**, 7-31.

Grotberg, E. (1975). Adjustment problems of the gifted. In W.B. Barbe and J.S. Renzulli (eds.). *Psychology and Education of the Gifted.* (London: John Wiley).

Guilford, J.P: (1950). Creativity. *American Psychologist,* **5**, 444-454

Halsey, A.H. (1977). Genetics, social structure and intelligence. In A.H. Halsey (ed.). *Heredity and Environment.* (London: Methuen).

Hargreaves, D.H. (1967). *Social Relations in a Secondary School.* (London: Routledge and Kegan Paul).

Hargreaves, D.H. (1972). *Interpersonal Relations and Education.* (London Routledge and Kegan Paul).

Hargreaves, D.H. (1972). *Interpersonal Relations and Education.* (London: R.K.P.).

Hargreaves, D.H. (1977). The process of typification in classroom interaction: models and methods. *British Journal of Educational Psychology,* **47**, 274-284.

Hargreaves, D.H., Hester, S.K. and Mellor, F.J. (1975). *Deviance in Classrooms.* (London: Routledge and Kegan Paul).

Harlow, H.F. (1969). Age-mate or peer affectional system. In D.S. Lerhman, R.A. Hinde and E. Shaw (eds.). *Advances in the Study of Behaviour,* **2,** (New York: Academic Press).

Hartup, W.W. and Lougee, M.D. (1975). Peer interactions. *School Psychologist,* **4,** 11-21.

Hasan, P. and Butcher, H.J. (1966). Creativity and intelligence, a partial replication with Scottish children of Getzels' and Jacksons' study. *British Journal of Psychology,* **57**, 129-135.

Herbert, J. (1967). *A System for Analysing Lessons.* (New York: Teachers College Press).

Herrnstein, R.J. (1973). *IQ in the Meritocracy.* (London: Allen Lane).

Hess, R.D. and Shipman, V.C. (1965). Early experience and the socialization of cognitive modes in children. *Child Development,* **36**, 869-86.

Hill, C. (1975). *The World Turned Upside Down: Radical Ideas during the English Revolution.* (Harmondsworth: Penguin).

Hitchfield, E.M. (1973). *In Search of Promise.* (London: Longman).

Hollingworth, L. (1942). *Children above 180 IQ.* (New York: Harcourt, Brace).

Holt, J. (1967). *How Children Fail.* (New York: Pitman).

Holt, J. (1969). *The Underachieving School.* (New York: Pitman).

Hopkinson, D. (1978). *The Education of Gifted Children.* (London: Woburn Press).

Hoyle, E. (1969). *The Role of the Teacher.* (London: Routledge and Kegan Paul).

Hoyle, E. and Wilks, J. (1975). *Gifted Children and Their Education.* (London: Department of Education and Science).

Hudson, L. (1966). *Contrary Imaginations.* (London: Methuen).

Hunt, J. McV. (1961). *Intelligence and Experience.* (New York: The Ronald Press).

Illich, I. (1970). *Deschooling Society.* (New York: Harper and Row).

Illingworth, R.S. (1964). *The Normal School Child.* (London: Heinemann Medical Books).

Insel, P.M. and Lindgren, H.C. (1978). *Too Close for Comfort: The Psychology of Crowding.* (New Jersey: Prentice Hall).

Jackson, Brian. (1964). *Streaming: An Education System in Miniature.* (London: Routledge and Kegan Paul).

Janeway, E. (1977). *Man's World, Woman's Place.* (London: Penguin).

Jencks, C. (1973). *Inequality.* (London: Allen Lane).

Jensen, A.R. (1972). *Genetics and Education.* (London: Methuen).

Jensen, A.R. (1973a). *Educational Differences.* (London: Methuen).

Jensen, A.R. (1973b). *Educability and Group Differences.* (London: Methuen).

Jones, Kathleen. (1972). *A History of the Mental Health Services.* (London: Routledge and Kegan Paul).

Kagan, J. and Moss, H.A. (1962). *Birth to Maturity.* (New York and London: John Wiley).

Kagan, J., Sontag, L.W., Baker, C.T. and Nelson, V.L. (1958). Personality and IQ change. *Journal of Abnormal and Social Psychology,* **56,** 261–266.

Kamin, Leon J. (1974). *The Science and Politics of IQ.* (New York: John Wiley).

Kernan, C.M. (1972). Language behaviour in a black urban community. *Monographs of the Language-Behaviour Research Laboratory, No. 2.* University of California.

Kipnis, D. McBride (1976). Intelligence, occupational status and achievement orientation. In J. Archer and B. Lloyd (eds.). *Exploring Sex Differences.* (London and New York: Academic Press).

Koestler, A. (1976). *The Thirteenth Tribe.* (London: Hutchinson).

Lasko, J.K. (1954). Parent behaviour towards first and second children. *Genetic Psychological Monographs,* **49,** 96–137. In Sutton-Smith and Rosenberg.

Lawick-Goodall, J. van (1971). *In the Shadow of Man.* (Glasgow: Collins).

Lawson, A. and Ingleby, J.D. (1974). Daily routines of preschool children: effects of age, birth order, sex and social class. *Psychological Medicine,* **4,** 399–415.

Lemert, E.M. (1951). *Social Pathology.* (New York: McGraw Hill).

Lenneberg, E.H. (1967). *Biological Foundations of Language.* (New York and London: John Wiley).

Lesley, C. (1976). *The Life of Noel Coward.* (London: Jonathan Cape).

Lorenz, K. (1966). *On Aggression.* (London: Methuen).

Love, L.R. and Kaswan, J.W. (1974). *Troubled Children: Their Families, Schools and Treatments.* (New York: John Wiley).

Lyon, Harold C. Jnr. (1976). Realising our potential. In Joy Gibson and Prue Chennells (eds.). *Gifted Children - Looking to their Future.* (London: Latimer).

McAskie, M. and Clarke, A.M. (1976). Parent offspring resemblances in intelligence: theories and evidence. *British Journal of Psychology,* **67,** 243–273.

McClelland, D.C. (1961). *The Achieving Society.* (Princeton, New Jersey: Van Nostrand).

McClelland, D.C., Atkinson, J.W., Clark, R.A. and Lowell, E.L. (1953). *The Achievement Motive.* (New York: Appleton-Century-Crofts).

Maccoby, E.E. (1966). Sex differences in intellectual functioning. In E.E. Maccoby (ed.). *The Development of Sex Differences.* (Stanford: Stanford University Press).

Maccoby, E.E. and Jacklin, C.N. (1974). *The Psychology of Sex Differences.* (Stanford: Stanford University Press).

Macfarlane, A. (1974). If a smile is so important. *New Scientist,* April.

MacKinnon, D.W. (1962). The personality correlates of creativity: a study of American architects. *Proceedings of the 14th Congress of Applied Psychology.* (Copenhagen: Munksgaard).

Mays, S. (1969). *Reuben's Corner.* (London: Pan Books).

Mays, J. (1973). Delinquent and maladjusted children. In V.P. Verma (ed.). *Stresses in Children.* (London: ULP).

Mercer, J.R. (1975). Psychological assessment and the rights of children. In N. Hobbs (ed.). *The Classification of Children,* Vol. 1. (San Francisco: Jossey-Bass).

# Bibliography

Meyer, R.J. and Haggerty, R.J. (1962). Streptococcal infections in families. *Paediatrics*, **29**, 539-49.

Miles, C.C. (1954). Gifted children. In L. Carmichael (ed.). *Manual of Child Psychology*. (New York: John Wiley).

Morrison, A. and McIntyre, D. (1969). *Teachers and Teaching*. (Harmondsworth: Penguin).

Morrison, A. and McIntyre, D. (1972). *Social Psychology of Teaching*. (London: Penguin).

Moss, H.A. and Kagan, J. (1961). Stability of achievement and recognition-seeking behaviour from early childhood through adulthood. *Journal of Abnormal and Social Psychology*, **63**, 504-513.

Mussen, P.H. and Jones, M.C. (1957). Self conceptions, motivations and interpersonal attitudes of late and early-maturing boys. *Child Development*, **29**, 61-67.

Mussen, P.H., Conger, J.J. and Kagan, J. (1969). *Child Development and Personality*. (New York: Harper and Row).

Myrdal, G. (1970). *Objectivity in Social Research*. (London: Duckworth).

Nelson, J.D., Gefland, D.M. and Hartmann, D.P. (1969). Children's aggression following competition and exposure to an aggressive model. *Child Development*, **40**, 1085-97.

Newbold, D. (1977). *Ability Grouping - The Banbury Enquiry*. (Windsor: NFER).

New Scientist. (1978). Maths in the sun. 3rd August.

Newson, J. and Newson, E. (1976). On the social origins of symbolic functioning. In P. Varma and P. Williams (eds.). *Advances in Educational Psychology III*. (London: Hodder and Stoughton).

Newson, J. and Newson, E. (1977). *Perspectives On School at Seven Years Old*. (London: George Allen and Unwin).

Nisbet, J. and Entwistle, J.J. (1967). Intelligence and size of family. *British Journal of Educational Psychology*, **37**, 2.

Oden, M. (1968). The fulfilment of promise: a 40 year follow-up of the Terman Gifted Group. *General Psychology Monthly*, **77**.

Ogilvie, E. (1973). *Gifted Children in Primary Schools*. (London and Basingstoke: Macmillan).

Painter, F. (1976). Research into attainment levels of gifted British primary school children. In J. Gibson and P. Chennells (eds.). *Gifted Children - Looking to their Future*. (London: Latimer).

Parkyn, G.W. (1976). The identification and evaluation of gifted children. In J. Gibson and P. Chennells, (eds.) *Gifted Children - Looking to their Future*. (London: Latimer).

Pasold, E.W. (1977 *Ladybird, Ladybird*. (Manchester: Manchester University Press).

Pavlov, I.P. (1927). *Conditioned Reflexes*. (New York: Dover).

Pegnato, C.W. and Birch, J.W. (1959). Locating gifted children in Junior High Schools. *Exceptional Children*, No. 25.

Peterson, D.R., Becker, W.C., Hellmer, L.A., Shoemaker, D.J. and Quay, H.C. (1959). Parental attitudes and child adjustment. *Child Development*, **30**, 119-130.

Phillips, C and Bannon, W.J. (1968). The Stanford-Binet Form L-M, 3rd revision. A local English study of norms, concurrent validity and social differences. *British Journal of Educational Psychology*, **38**, 148-161.

Piaget, J. (1968). *The Moral Judgement of The Child*. (London: Routledge and Kegan Paul).

Piaget, J. (1971). *Structuralism*. (London: Routledge and Kegan Paul).

Pilling, D. and Pringle, M.L.K. (1978). *Controversial Issues in Child Development*. (London: Elek).

Porter, R.B. and Cattell, R.B. (1959). *Handbook for the IPAT Children's Personality Questionnaire*. (Champaign, Ill: IPAT)

Postman and Weingartner. (1975). *Teaching as a Subversive Activity*. (Harmondsworth: Penguin).

Potter, Stephen. (1950). *Lifemanship*. (London: Rupert Hart-Davis).

Povey, R.M. (1975). Educating the gifted. *Journal of the Association of Educational Psychologists*, **3**, 9.

Pringle, M.L.K. (1966). *Social Learning and its Measurement*. (London: Longmans).

Pringle, M.L.K. (1970). *Able Misfits*. (London: Longmans).

Pringle, M.L.K., Butler, N.R. and Davie, R. (1966). *11,000 Seven Year Olds*. (London: Longmans).

Rapoport, Rhona and Rapoport, Robert. (1971). *Dual Career Families*. (London: Penguin).

Rapoport, R., Rapoport, R. and Strelitz, Z.'(1977). *Fathers, Mothers and Others*. (London: Routledge and Kegan Paul).

Raven, J.C. (1965). *Guide to Using the Coloured Progressive Matrices*. (London: H.K. Lewis).

Raven, J. (1977). *Education, Values and Society*. (London: H.K. Lewis; New York: The Psychological Corporation).

Renvoize, J. (1975). *Children in Danger*. (London: Penguin).

Revesz, G. (1953). *An Introduction to the Psychology of Music*. (London: Longmans).

Roff, M. and Sells, S.B. (1968). Juvenile delinquency in relation to peer acceptance-rejection and socio-economic status. *Psychology in the Schools*, **5**, 3-18.

Roget, Peter Mark. (1962). *Roget's Thesaurus of English Words and Phrases*. (London: Longmans).

Rosenthal, R. and Jacobson, L. (1968). *Pygmalion in the Classroom*. (New York: Holt).

Rowlands, P. (1964). *Gifted Children and their Problems*. (London: J.M. Dent).

Rutter, M. (1965). Classification and categorisation in child psychiatry. *Journal of Child Psychology and Psychiatry*, **6**, 71-83.

Rutter, M. (1971). Parent-child separation; psychological effects on the children. *Journal of Child Psychology and Psychiatry*, **12**, 233.

Rutter, M. (1972). *Maternal Deprivation Reassessed*. (Harmondsworth: Penguin).

Rutter, M., Quinton, D. and Yule, W. (1976).·*Family Pathology And Disorder In The Children*. (London: John Wiley).

Rutter, M., Tizard, J. and Whitmore, K. (1970). *Education Health and Behaviour*. (London: Longmans).

Rutter, M., Yule, B., Quinton, D., Rowlands, O., Yule, W. and Berger, M. (1974). Attainment and adjustment in two geographical areas. III. *British Journal of Psychiatry*, **125**, 520-33.

Sapir, E. (1929). The status of linguistics as a science. *Language*, **5**, 207-214.

Selg, J. (1975). *The Making of Human Aggression*. (London: Quartet Books).

Schaffer, H.R. (1974). Behavioural synchrony in infancy. *New Scientist*, **4**.

Shields, J.B. (1968). *The Gifted Child*. (Windsor: NFER).

Shipman, M.D. (1972). *The Limitations of Social Research*. (London: Longmans).

Shuter, Rosamund. (1968). *The Psychology of Musical Ability*. (London: Methuen).

Silberman, C.E. (1970). *Crisis in the Classroom*. (New York: Random House).

Skinner, B.F. (1953). *Science and Human Behaviour*. (New York: Macmillan).

Stanley, J.C. (ed.). (1973). *Compensatory Education for Children ages 2-8: Recent Studies of Educational Intervention*. (Baltimore: John Hopkins University Press).

Stanley, Julian C., Keating, Daniel P. and Fox, Lynn H. (1974). *Mathematical Talent: Discovery, Description and Development*. (London and Baltimore: Johns Hopkins University Press).

Stein, A.H. and Bailey, M.M. (1973). The socialisation of achievement orientation in females. *Psychological Bulletin*, **80**, 345-66.

Stein, Z., Susser, M., Saenger, G. and Marrolla, F. (1975). *Famine and Human Develop-*

# Bibliography

*ment: the Dutch Hunger Winter of 1944-1945.* (New York: Oxford University Press).

Steinman, R. and Traunstein, D. (1976). Reducing deviance: the self-help challenge to the human services. *Journal of Applied Behavioural Science,* **12,** 347.

Stott, D.H. (1976). *The Social Adjustment of Children.* (London: Hodder and Stoughton).

Stott, M.B. (1945). Some differences between boys and girls in vocational guidance. *Occupational Psychology,* **19,** 121-131.

Sutton-Smith, B. and Rosenberg, B.G. (1970). *The Siblings.* (New York: Holt, Rinehart & Winston).

Sutton-Smith, B. and Rosenberg, B.G. (1970). *The Siblings.* (New York: Holt).

Tanner, J.M. (1974). Variability in growth and maturity in new-born infants. In M. Lewis and L.A. Rosenblum (eds.). *The Effect of the Infant on its Caregivers.* (New York: John Wiley).

Tanner, J.M. (1978). *Foetus into Man.* (London: Open Books).

Tempest, N.R. (1974). *Teaching Clever Children, 7-11.* (London: Routledge and Kegan Paul).

Terman, L.M. (1925). *Genetic Studies of Genius - Vol. 1. Mental and Physical Traits of a Thousand Gifted Children.* (California: Stanford University Press).

Terman, L.M. and Merrill, M.A. (1961). *Stanford-Binet Intelligence Scale. Manual for the third revision Form I-M.* (London: Harrap).

Terman, L.M. and Oden, M. (1959). *The Gifted Group at Mid-Life. Genetic Studies of Genius.* (Stanford: Stanford University Press).

Terman, L.M. (1925). *Genetic Studies of Genius - Vol. 1. Mental and Physical Traits of a Thousand Gifted Children.* (California: Stanford University Press).

Thorndike, R.L. (1968). Review of Pygmalion in the Classroom by Rosenthal and Jacobson. *AERA Journal,* 5, 4.

Tizard, J., Moss, P. and Perry, J. (1976). *All Our Children.* (London: Temple Smith).

Torrance, E.P. (1962). Developing creative thinkings through school experiences. In S.F. Parnes and H.F. Harding (eds.), *A Source Book for Creative Thinkings* (New York: Scribner).

Torrance, E.P. (1965). *Rewarding Creative Behaviour.* (Englewood Cliffs, N.J; Prentice-Hall).

Torrance, E.P. (1969). Prediction of adult creative achievement among high school seniors. *Gifted-Child Quarterly,* **13**

Torrance, E.P. (1975). Emerging concepts of giftedness. In W.B. Barber and J.S. Renzulli (eds.). *Psychology and Education of the Gifted.* (New York: John Wiley).

Tousley, A.E. (1967). *Reading and Remedial Reading.* (London: Routledge and Kegan Paul).

Tulkin, S.R. and Kagan, J. (1972). Mother-child interaction in the first year of life. *Child Development,* **43,** 31-41.

Turner, R.H. (1964). Some aspects of women's ambitions. *American Journal of Sociology,* **70,** 271-285.

Vernon, P.E. (1955). The assessment of children. *Studies in Education, No. 7.* (London: Institute of Education).

Vernon, P.E. (1957). *Secondary School Selection.* (London: Methuen).

Vernon, P.E. (1961). *The Structure of Human Abilities.* (London: Methuen).

Vernon, P.E., Adamson, G. and Vernon, D. (1977). *The Psychology and Education of Gifted Children.* (London: Methuen).

Wallach, M.A. and Kogan, N. (1965). *Modes of Thinking in Young Children: A Study of the Creativity-Intelligence Distinction.* (New York: Holt, Rinehart Winston).

Ward, J.S. (1975). Basic concepts. In W.B. Barbe and J.S. Renzulli (eds.). *Psychology and Education of the Gifted.* (London: John Wiley).

Watson, J.B. (1925). *Behaviourism.* (New York: Norton).

Wechsler, D. (1939). *The Measurement of Adult Intelligence.* (Baltimore: Williams and Wilkins).

Wechsler, D. (1949a). *Wechsler Intelligence Scale for Children.* (New York: Psychological Corporation).

Wechsler, D. (1949b). *Manual, Wechsler Intelligence Scale for Children.* (New York: Psychological Corporation).

Wing, J.K. (1978). *Reasoning About Madness.* (London: Oxford University Press).

Winick, M. (1971). Cellular growth during early malnutrition. *Paediatrics,* **47,** 969–78.

Winter, W.D. and Ferreira, A.J. (1969). *Research in Family Interaction: Readings and Commentary.* (Palo Alto, California: Science and Behaviour Books Inc.).

Wiseman, S. (1964). *Education and Environment.* (Manchester: Manchester University Press).

Woolf, V. (1978). *Moments of Being.* (Herts: Triad Panther).

Wooton, A.J. (1974). Talk in the homes of young children. *Sociology,* **8,** 277.

Wyndham, J. (1969). *The Midwich Cuckoos.* (Harmondsworth: Penguin).

Young, D. (1966). *Non Readers Intelligence Test.* (London: University of London Press).

Zax, M. and Cowen, E.L. (1969). Research on early detection and prevention of emotional dysfunction in young school children. In C.D. Spielberger (ed.). *Current Topics in Clinical and Community Psychology, Vol. 1.* (New York: Academic Press).

Zigler, E. and Butterfield, E.C. (1968). Motivational aspects of changes in IQ test performance of culturally deprived nursery school children. *Child Development,* **39,** 1–14.

# Index

abilities,
  assessment of, 79–82
  development of, 23
  differences between social groups, 62–9
  foreign language, 81
  inheritance of, 22
  musical and artistic, 68–9, 79, 152
    tests of, 80, 138
  physical, 69, 81
  verbal, as measure of socio-economic class, 66–7
abnormality, medical model of, 9–13
  limitations of, 12–13
acceleration, of gifted children, 264
achievement, 1, 31, 232–3
  assessment of, 88–95
  distinction from potential, 17
  orientation, 32–7
    sex differences in, 35–7
  *see* pupil achievement, teacher achievement
adjustment, of children, 120–2
  in Gulbenkian Project, 193–203
aggression,
  as learned behaviour, 127–8
  coping with, 47
anti-social disorders, *see* disorders
assessment,
  benefits and disadvantages of, 95
  continuous, 95
  in practice, 90–2
  large scale, problems of, 91
Assessment of Performance Unit (APU), 94
attention range, 159

babies, human,
  dialogue with mothers, 39
  sensitivity of, very early, 39–41
Bandura, A., *see* modelling
behaviour,
  disorders of, 122–3
  modification techniques, 129

behaviour (*cont.,*)
  normal, check lists for, 12
behaviourism, 22
birth,
  alertness at, 221
  and mother's age, relation to giftedness, 239–40
birth order, effect on intellect and personality, 41–4
birthweight, effect on later abilities, 73
books, availability as guide to reading attainment, 67
boredom at school, of gifted children, 241
Brentwood Experiment, 267
Bristol Social Adjustment Guides (BSAG), 136, 193
  *see* Gulbenkian Project
British Intelligence Scales, 103–4, 259

children, handicapped, 49
  in ordinary schools, 57
cognition (knowingness), 21, 26
comprehensive education,
  criticism of, 8
  founding of, 255
concentration, of gifted children, 231
conditioning,
  operant, 24
  reinforcement, 24–5
  theories on, limitations of, 25
conduct disorders, 122–3
co-ordination, in gifted children, 229–30
Coward, Noel, 11
creativity,
  and stability, 118
  concept of, 116–17
  schemes to promote, 117
  tests of, 120
curiosity, as indicator of giftedness, 227–8
curriculum,
  enrichment of, 266–8

curriculum (*cont.,*)
  open and hidden, 92
delinquency, 120-1
depression, among mothers, 50
deprivation, maternal, 85-6
deviance,
  and normality, 56-8
  primary, 57
  secondary, 58
  *see also* abnormality, labelling
disorders, anti-social, 122-3
  *see* behaviour, conduct disorders, neurotic
    disorders

Education Act (1944), 285-6
education,
  in industrial societies, 125-6
  relation with measured intelligence, 114
  selective, 255-61
    problems and benefits of, 259-61
  special, for gifted children, 91, 254-9
  *see also* study, independent, teachers and
    teaching, mixed ability
eleven-plus,
  as predictor of success, 116
  introduction of, 8, 255
  margin of error in, 256
energy, mental and physical, of gifted children,
  228-9
envionment, cultural, effect on learning, 55
  *see also* adjustment
excellence, criteria of, 88
expectancy effect, 61-2

family,
  communication in, 37
  discordant, 48-52
  problem behaviour of children in, 49
  size of, effect on children, 41-4
  socialization in, 37-44
first-born, prevalence among gifted, 153-4
friendships,
  as indicator of development, 45
  effect on children, 44-8
  of gifted children, 157, 238

genius, and psychiatric abnormalities, 9
gifted children,
  achievements, assessment of, 88
  beneficial methods of education for, 11
  birth order and family size, effects of, 41-4
  boys, difficulty with, 30-1
  disturbed behaviour among, 51
  economic value of, 19
  educational needs of, 277-9
  effect of socio-economic class on, 63-4, 66, 84
  feelings of difference of, 237-8
  friendships of, 44-8

gifted children (*cont.,*)
  identification of, 13-17
  in schools, 11-12
  interests of, 228
  maladjustment in, 124-5
  problems of, 250-4
  role of, 30
  selection of, 10
  self-concept of, 238, 247-50
  sexes, ratio between, 32
  social interaction of, 27
  traditional views of, 3-5
  *see also* Gulbenkian Project, research
    methods, teaching, teachers
giftedness,
  definition of, 3
  dependence on social values and culture,
    1
  developmental evidence of, early, 221-3
    general, 223-33
  difference from achievement, 1
  in English, forms of, 80
  judging, 71
  meaning of, 1-19
  measured by IQ, 2-3
  mythology of, 5-9, 87
    dispelling of, 241-3
    influence in development of English
      educational system, 8
  problems of, 11-13
girls, early maturing of, 84-5
grammar schools, introduction of, 8, 255
groups, social, 28
Gulbenkian Project on gifted children, 131-214
  basis of, 131
  control and target groups,
    investigation of, 143-63
    selection of, 132-5
    summary of, 167-9
  data, collection of, 140
  design of, 135-6
  headteachers of schools in, 206-10
  health of children in, 163-4, 186-8, 198
  measures used in, 136-40
  ratio of sexes in, 201
  results of, 146-63
  review of, 216-20
  schools in, types of, 203-6
  *see* IQ groups

halo effect, 62
Head Start Program (USA), 85
health,
  mental and physical, relation between, 77
  of gifted children, 224-5
  *see* Gulbenkian Project
height, relationship with mental ability, 75
hostility in children, development of, 127-8

humour, sense of, and gifted children, 250

independence, and gifted children, 236-7
intellectual achievement, and short-
    sightedness, 226
intelligence,
    and achievement, relationship between, 83
    as measured by test, 65
    children's, and father's occupational status,
        66
    fresh concepts of, 103-4
    genetic component in, 64
    measures of, 104-13
    models of, 79
    sex differences in, 113-16
    *see also* IQ tests
IQ groups in Gulbenkian Project, 169-98,
        202-3
    comparisons in target group, 184-6
    health in, 186-8
    high and moderate, 172-84
    summary of, 191-2
IQ tests,
    applied to different races, 101-2, 109
    as measure of giftedness, 2-3, 14, 79
    make up of, 110-13
    minimum for entry to grammar school, 256
    verbal bias of, 100
    *see also* Raven's progressive matrices,
        Stanford-Binet intelligence tests,
        Wechsler intelligence scales

kibbutz, multiple mothering in, 46-7

labelling,
    as cause of bad behaviour, 61
    as response of society, 59
    effect of, 58
learning experiences, early, 85-7
    overestimation of importance, 86
    skills of, assessment, 90
learning techniques, acquisition of, 271

maladjustment of children, 120-1, 234-6
    seeking help for, 128-9
    sources of, 123-8
mathematical abilities, connection with verbal
        abilities, 81
memory, of gifted children, 231
middle class, sunken, 257
modelling, 25-7, 48, 52
Montessori method of infant learning, 87
mother-baby dialogue, 39
    class differences in, 64
Munch, Edward, 9
musical abilities, *see* abilities
mythology, social, 5, 13
    *see also* gifted children

National Association for Gifted Children (UK),
        13, 20, 51, 68, 132, 216-18, 273-5
    reasons for membership of, 166-7
National Children's Bureau, 52
National Merit Scholarship Program (USA),
        19
nature-nurture controversy, 22
neurotic disorders, 122-3
Nijinsky, 9
normality, 56-62, 121-2
    *see also* deviance
nursery education,
    demand for, 85
    value for gifted children, 46

one-parent families, 51-2

parent-teacher associations, 207-8
peer relationships, importance of, 45-8
personality, development of, 233-8
physical development of children, 72-9
    and mental ability, 75-7
    before birth, 72-4
    difficulties of description, 72
    sexual differences, 74-5
Piaget, J., 47, 65
Plato, 3
play, pattern of, 239
potential of children,
    judging, 82-7
    prediction of, 83
    *see* IQ tests
private schools, growth of, 255-6
project work in primary schools, 264
psychological counselling in schools, 208-9
psychology, development of, 9
    educational, in teacher training programme,
        268-9
punishment, 49
pupil achievement, importance of assessment
        of, 93-4

Raven's progressive matrices, 107-8
    ceiling effect in, 145
reading skills of gifted children, 222-3
research methods on gifted children
    confirmation, 102-3
    design, 99-100
    interpretation, 100-2
    problems of, 96-103
    selection, 96-8
    *see* Gulbenkian Project

roles social, 29-32

Russia,
    selection system for gifted children, 98
    schools in, comparison with American
        schools, 126

schools,
    assessment in, 92–6
    happiness of children in, 158
    influence on children of, 52–5
    research in, 53
    state and private, comparisons between, 210–14
    stress among pupils in, 125–7
secondary modern schools, introduction and role of, 255–6
self-evaluation, importance of, 95
self-help groups, 273–5
sensitivity, of gifted children, 240–1
sleep cycles, 122, 164
    of gifted children, 156, 188, 223–4
social differences, 62–9
social interaction, theories of, 27
social learning, 25, 51
    early, effectiveness of, 85
    intervention of cognition in, 27
social skills, IQ as a predictor of, 41
socialization, 21, 25
    in schools, 52–5
    in the family, 37–44
    processes, 28–37
    two-way, 38–9
socio-economic class, effect of, 63–4
sport, relationship with giftedness, 158–9
Stanford–Binet intelligence test, 104–5, 136
    correlation with Wechsler intelligence scales, 105
    make-up of, 111
Stanley, Professor Julian, 36
stature, physical, of gifted children, 225
stomach complaints in children, 78

study, independent,
    criticisms of, 265
    for gifted children, 264

talents, of gifted children, 2
talking, early, as sign of giftedness, 222
TAT test, 33
teachers,
    achievement of, research into, 92–3
    as parents of gifted children, 165–6, 190, 200
    attitudes, effect of, 269–70
    centres, 267
    training of, 268–70
teaching,
    formal, comparison to informal, 102
    gifted children, 270
    in comprehensive schools, 262
    mixed ability, 261
    styles of, 272
team teaching, 265
technical schools, introduction and role of, 255
testing, pluralistic, 60
thinking skills, critical, assessment of, 90
twins, IQ of, 101

understanding of gifted children, 231–2

Van Gogh, Vincent, 9
verbal abilities, *see* abilities, IQ tests

walking, early, as sign of giftedness, 221–2
Warnock report, 94, 227
Wechsler intelligence scales, 105–7
    make up of, 112
World Council for Gifted Children, 19
Woolf, Virginia, 6, 9